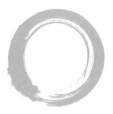

FACIAL GUA SHA:
A STEP-BY-STEP GUIDE TO A NATURAL FACELIFT

Clive Witham

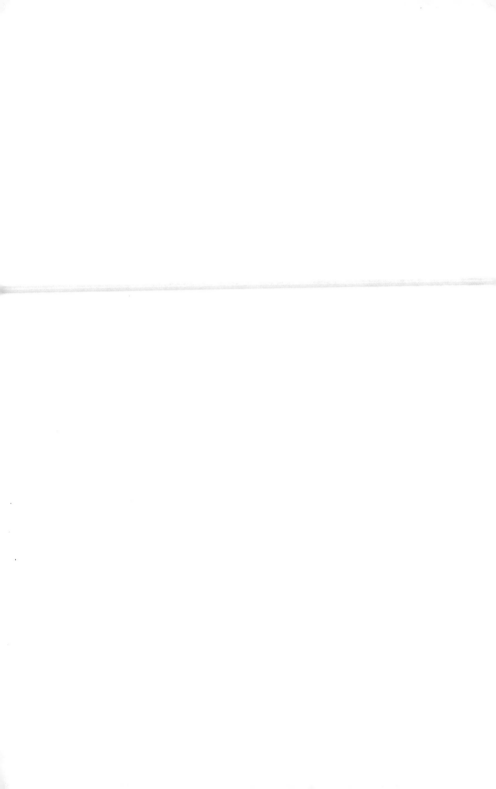

Published in Jan 2018 by Mangrove Press, UK.

ISBN: 978-0-9561507-6-9

Mangrove Press
Martello House
2 Western Road
Poole, UK

Disclaimer: The information in this book is given in good faith and is neither intended to diagnose any physical or mental condition nor to serve as a substitute for informed medical advice or care.

Please contact your health professional for medical advice and treatment. Neither the author nor the publisher can be held liable by any person for any loss or damage whatsoever which may arise from the use of this book or any of the information herein.

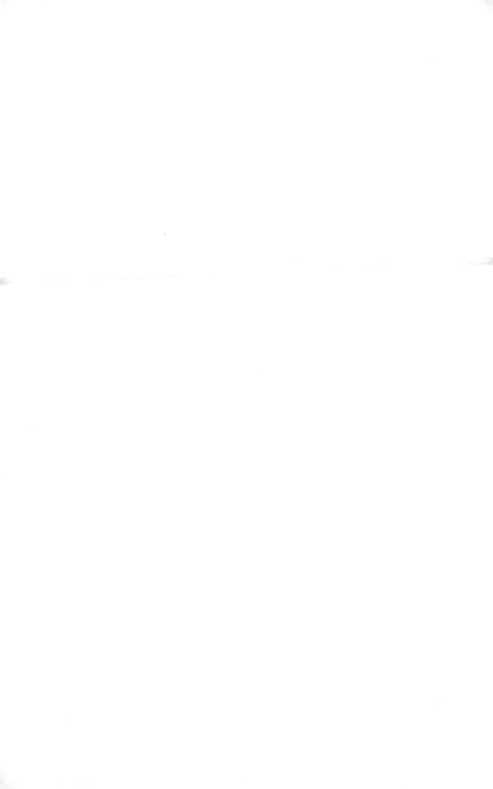

CONTENTS

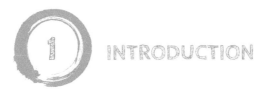

1 INTRODUCTION

BEAUTY IS BUSINESS

Let us start with some facts.

○ There are more than 20 million cosmetic procedures carried out worldwide every year and the number is growing substantially year upon year[1].

○ Most of these procedures take place in four countries: the USA, Brazil, South Korea and Japan.

○ Four million of these 20 million treatments are face and head procedures such as facelifts and eyelid surgery, and around 7 million are Botox injections.

So, with facelifts at around $6,000 and Botox treatments between $200 to $500 a-time, clearly large sums of money are changing hands in the pursuit of beauty. But more than the jaw-dropping amounts of money involved, the worrying thing is why are so many people so intent on changing their faces.

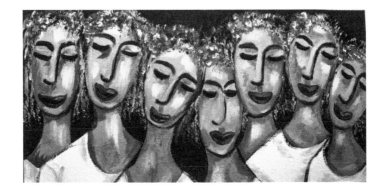

THE EGYPTIANS

The search for beauty is nothing new. It has been going on for thousands of years and involved all sorts of remedies both familiar and strange. Four thousand years ago, the ancient Egyptians were using animal oils, copper flakes, salt, earth, fish glue (that is gelatine made from the bladders of sturgeon fish in case you are wondering), vinegar and alabaster to improve skin texture[2]. They had decided that an ideal face contained many rounded features such as a rounded, short nose, rounded chin, sloping forehead and thick lips.

THE GREEKS

While these features dominated the artful representation of Egyptian Pharaohs for millennia, the ancient Greeks decided to go one step further and mathematically calculate the correct facial proportions of beauty. They did this by deciding that the face should be divided into three sections: From the hairline to the eyes; from the eyes to the upper lip; and from the upper lip to the chin. For beauty to be established, the three sections had to be equal in height.

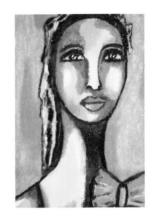

To this they added that the width of the face had to be in correct proportion to its length. To calculate exactly how big this proportion was, they drew on great philosophers and mathematicians like Plato (428 – 347 BCE) and Euclid (365 – 300 BCE) and applied the idea of the Golden Ratio - also known as 'phi' after the 21st letter of the Greek alphabet - to the face. This meant that the length of the face should be 1.618 times the width, and width in turn should be 0.618 times the length. And so beauty had a number.

These ancient ideas stuck in the western world and feature greatly in art and sculpture especially from the renaissance period (1300 – 1600 CE) onwards. Leonardo da Vinci's Mona Lisa is a classic example of the proportions of the golden ratio.

THE CHINESE

The ancient Chinese also had a stab at defining what it means to be beautiful. Cosmetic treatments known as 'Mei Rong' can be dated all the way back to the Qin Dynasty (221-206 BCE) where herbs and acupuncture were used to try and preserve the youth and beauty of the court concubines[3].

They had a similar idea in dividing the face into three equal horizontal sections but they differed in the landmarks to do it: From the hairline to the eyebrows; from the eyebrows to the bottom of the nose; and from the bottom of the nose to the chin.

The width of the face was divided into five equal parts, each the width of an eye. This classification was called 'three stops and five eyes' and later became known as the vertical thirds and horizontal fifths rule[4].

BEYOND CALCULATIONS

The fact that beauty has been mathematically quantified is fine as an academic exercise but does not however take into account that we see life through different eyes. What represents beauty for one person may not represent beauty for another. Indeed it should not take you too long to think of someone who is generally regarded as beautiful but who does not fit into these proportions[5] and anyway the whole exercise becomes rather redundant when you realize the fact that virtually no one actually has these proportions in the real world[6].

THE BEAUTY WITHIN

Beauty is therefore more about our perceptions of the world around us than any social norm. And this perception comes from our own emotional-psychological make-up that we bring with us to any perceived preference. To put it in other words, our own beauty and those of others is a direct reflection of our emotional, physical, mental, spiritual state inside our own bodies. Despite what we are bombarded with on a daily basis through media channels, it is not the sum reflection of the first layer of skin that surrounds your body and the muscles and bones that support it. We are essentially who we are inside. Not outside. Beauty shows itself when the internal balance of your body is at its optimum level and what is inside quite literally radiates outwards.

A NATURAL SOLUTION

Which brings me to the point
of this book. It is not about getting a quick fix. It is not about the
latest cosmetic fad. It is not about
changing to what other people
tell you that you should be. It is
all about enhancing who you are.
How you look. Both inside and
outside. It is about how the present and the past has impacted on
making you the person reading
this right now. It is about using
that information and bridging
the gap, either perceived or real,
between the past you and the
present you. The natural facelift
in the title is referring not only
to the cosmetic idea of changes
at the skin level but equally at
changing the face we show to the
outside world. An external and
internal facelift. In this way it
can help to lift the veil which can
often obscure the real you.

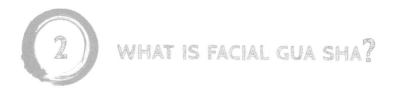

2 WHAT IS FACIAL GUA SHA?

SCRAPING YOUR SKIN

In China, where Gua sha is used as part of treatments to reduce the effects of aging and enhance the skin, it is claimed that regular facial Gua sha can promote the growth of new skin cells, help renew your complexion and reduce clogged pores, control acne, tighten the chin and enhance the ability of your skin to absorb make-up products[7]. You may be wondering how the simple action of scraping the skin without any special creams or oils or lotions or ointments or cleansing milks or serums or masks or magical ingredients of any kind, can actually do anything close to this. Perhaps you are thinking that it is in fact a superficial beauty fad, created out of thin air to make someone super rich. After all, in facial Gua sha, all that occurs is you drag a blunt flat object along the skin of your face, head, neck and other areas of the body to stimulate your skin. That blunt object may be an expensive state of the art Gua sha board or it may be a simple Chinese soup spoon. You can spread your face with the latest beauty products for lubrication or you can just use any face oil.

HEALTH REALITIES

You may also be wondering that if it is so cheap and effective, why you have not heard much about it before. Well, that would be a very good question. I specialise in health education and promotion and it is quite frankly astonishing how often the simple things that cost so little are overlooked in favour of heavily publicised products and treatments promoted by huge multinational companies and the pursuit of the contents of your wallet. Sometimes you just need to take a step back and ignore the constant bombardment of the beauty business, in favour of something that does not have tanned doctors with shiny white teeth giving their stamp of approval on some concoction which has just been created in a puff of smoke in their laboratory.

MORE THAN SCRAPING

So with Gua sha, all you are doing is dragging a Gua sha tool across your skin, right?

No, I have to admit I misled you slightly. That may actually be your action and what it might look like to anyone watching. But facial Gua sha is far more than this and in this section we will look at what happens to your skin when you do facial Gua sha.

BLOOD AND OXYGEN

The essence of how Gua sha treats the face and the body is in the flow of blood and oxygen. The ancient Chinese had a sophisticated understanding of how blood and oxygen move around the body. You may have come across the word Qi. It is commonly used in Oriental medicine and essentially refers to the idea of nourishing the body with a constant flow of oxygenated blood full of nutrients. If this flow is normal then your body is functioning well but when not, your body will react and send signals in the form of pain, stiffness, discomfort etc.

SKIN CHANGES

The idea with facial Gua sha is either to prevent or support changes in the blood flow in the muscles and tissues of your facial area. The action of Gua sha can make immediate changes to the colour of the skin. When done more vigorously on the body, this change produces what might be petechiae (pe-tee-kiya), which are small red dots bunched together and which resemble a rash (see image 1). This is when the tissue bed releases blood and it gets trapped in the extravascular space under the skin[8]. This is the meaning of the 'sha' in 'Gua sha'. It is referring, among other things, to these dots on the skin, while 'Gua' means to scrape. For facial Gua sha, it is generally not a good idea for these petechiae or sha to appear on the surface of the skin. They usually appear when Gua sha is applied with a strong technique to the body. For the face, however, the technique is much gentler and rather than the short, pressured scrapes used to treat your body, you sweep (not scrape) the tool in one smooth movement. After a few sweeps, the skin which you swept over will usually go pinkish but no sign of petechiae.

12

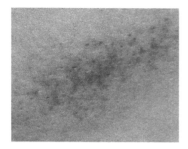

Image 1: petechiae

BLOOD FLOW CHANGES

The reason the skin changes, whether it be a slight pink hue in facial Gua sha or full-on petechiae in body Gua sha, is that the action of Gua sha on the surface of the skin increases blood flow to that area. Indeed, Gua sha is thought to make changes in subcutaneous micro-vascular pressure which causes the blood vessels to dilate and which increases not only the flow of blood but also the temperature in the local area[9].

AREAS OF CHANGE

While you can do Gua sha anywhere with muscle or tissue underneath the skin to increase this local blood flow, there are actually areas and channels throughout your face and body where this change is much more profound. Research has demonstrated that the heat produced in the tissues, known as thermal conductivity, is more remarkable when applying Gua sha along established Chinese medicine channels than on other parts of the body[10]. This means that if you can follow the particular Chinese paths mapped out over generation upon generation as having an effect on the musculature, Gua sha will be more effective.

You may notice as you work your way through this book that I mention channels a great deal. You will see all kinds of illustrations with coloured lines snaking their way over the body and I will give instructions to scrape along this line and that line. Well, this is the reason. You can scrape anywhere and help your body out, but scrape on the correct channel for any given issue and it will work so much better. This is about replacing the idea of mediocre, superficial changes with real, tangible rejuvenation. If you use Gua sha without the theory of how it works, you will have to settle for the former. If you follow the relationships of how your body is connected to and reflected in your face, you are heading for the latter.

So far, we have established two important points. If you apply Gua sha, blood and nutrient

13

flow will improve in your muscles and tissues and if you follow particular lines, you can actually increase that flow even more. There is, however, even more to facial Gua sha than this and to illustrate the point let me turn to the natural world and plants.

THE ROOT

If the muscles in your face do not have a constant supply of this oxygen- and nutrient-rich blood, they will wither over time much like the leaves of a plant. I know to my cost that if I forget to water the plant which sits patiently in my clinic, its leaves begin to die and go brown at the edges. The cause of the problem is, of course, not in the leaf but in the soil in the plant pot and the stem's ability to absorb moisture. If I did not know much about the workings of a plant (which I do not), I might choose to water the leaf because clearly to me the plant looks fine, so the problem must be in the leaf. I could water the leaf and perhaps it may appear more moist and shiny for a while, but it would only be a matter of time before it began to wither again. And then more leaves would start withering. So I water them. They look fine for a while but again they are not healthy. I could then clip the leaf to take off the browning edges or I could snip them all off and hope to grow fresh ones. Meanwhile the stem is still dying and the soil is as dry as a desert.

My fixation on the leaf has meant that I ignored the rest of the plant and how the rest of the plant can change how the leaf looks and feels. Watering the soil and tending to the roots and stem of the plant would allow the moisture and nutrients to rise up and nourish each leaf. This natural process would not change the essential shape of the leaf because that is the type of plant it is, it will however give it life again. It will enhance its colour and texture and make it strong and healthy.

Perhaps at this point you can see the metaphor. Your face is part of your body and if you fixate on changing your face without acknowledging the influence the state of your body has over your face, as with the plant, your changes are not going to last very long. This is why many cosmetic operations have to be repeated. Your body wants to return to the same state that created the cosmetic features because the issue that caused them was never resolved.

TREAT THE WHOLE

It is for this reason that with Gua sha, it is important to not just treat your facial area but your head and your neck and your arms and legs. As mentioned earlier, research tells us that if Gua sha is done along the correct channels in your body, the result will be much more profound. This has always been the approach of Chinese cosmetology since ancient times: The close connection of facial appearance with the state of your internal organs, channels and blood[11].

So it is the state of the skin on the outside which is a reflection of the state of your body inside and this is the key to any effective beauty treatment. It must treat you on many levels: physically, mentally, even spiritually.

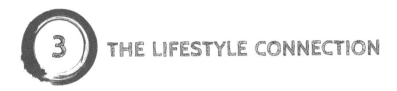

THE LIFESTYLE CONNECTION

In order to see your face in terms of the rest of the body, you have to reassess how your body has affected your face. Factors like smoking, a poor diet, a lack of exercise, overworking and under sleeping would have to be addressed as, if your body is at all weak, under-nourished or exhausted, it is going to show it on your skin.

NATURAL AGING

Before getting too far into lifestyle, it is important to clarify that there are many aspects of changes to your skin that you have no control over as you age. Your skin will change over time due to the reduction in elastic fibres and dermal bulk which will make your skin thinner, drier and more lax. It is perfectly normal and try as you may, you can delay it, but you cannot avoid it.

TISSUE

○ The connective tissue under your skin is made up of cells and protein fibres in a syrupy mixture known as 'ground substance'.

○ The most common type of fibres are collagen fibres and as we age these fibres increase in size and number and together with elastic fibres, cross link making them much less flexible and easy to fragment and lose shape.

○ The amount of water in the surrounding ground substance also drops which makes the fibres denser and restricts the movement of cells and substances from moving through the tissue. This means that less nutrients are available to supply the tissue.

The above two changes drastically reduce the elasticity of the skin and can lead to wrinkles.

SKIN

○ The top layers of your skin become thinner because the cells which usually are active in multiplying and replacing other cells (known as basal cells) become less active.

○ There are also often changes in the pigmentation of your skin due to a disruption in melanin production. Melanocytes, which are the cells that produce melanin, decrease in number steadily as we get older, making your skin paler. Some of the remaining melanocytes overproduce melanin causing age spots form on the skin's surface.

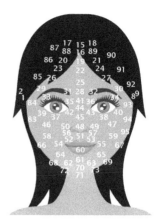

Image 2: Face Mapping

BONE AND CARTILAGE

○ Your nose and ear cartilage are less affected by the aging process and appear larger with age either due to continued growth or because of the loss of tissue mass in the rest of the face make them appear larger.

○ Bone mass reduces and cells called osteoclasts begin to break down more tissue in bones than are being created, causing them to lose some of their shape.

Changes of these kinds are totally out of your hands and are influenced by your genetics, ethnicity, hormones and physiological changes. Your lifestyle can make these changes more pronounced, but they would be there anyway no matter how you led your life.

FACE MAPPING

The ancient Chinese saw the face as one of the main health beacons of your body. They believed that it showed all manner of things related to the state of your health and wellbeing, so much so, that they developed facial mapping ideas which meant that your whole life, year by year, was quite literally on your face (see image 2).

Horizontal lines or distinctive marks would be interpreted as the face showing a traumatic event that happened around the age that the area of the face represents. The idea is that you can retrace major events in your life from the markings on your face. Image 2 shows the ages that correspond to that part of the face but note that for the ancient Chinese, you were already one years old when you were born, so you need to subtract one to correctly arrive at your age[12]. Also note that the facial number arrangement for men varies slightly but the focus here is not actually on the positioning of numbers but the fact that this idea that what happens in your life directly impacts your face, exists.

INDUCED AGING

While you have little control over traumatic or stressful events which may have created lines on your face, other causes of aging are in theory at least more under our control.

1. SUN

By far the most important lifestyle factor for your face is exposure to ultraviolet radiation either from the sun or artificial light. When this exposure directly causes skin change, it is referred to as photoaging and can be classified according to an established set of measures. This is known as the Glogau classification of skin photoaging which puts us into four different skin groups according to the severity of skin characteristics:

○ Mild: This typically refers to people in their late-20s/early-30s at only the initial stages of

photoaging when there are only minor pigment changes and no wrinkles.

○ Moderate: This is a much wider age group from people in their mid-30s to 50 with clearly established photoaging signs such as dynamic wrinkles, smile lines, the first signs of brown pigment changes.

○ Advanced: For the 50-65 year age group, the wrinkles have become static, discolourations of the skin are more prominent and spider veins develop.

○ Severe: The over 65s now have widespread wrinkles, skin malignancies, furrows and a yellow or grey skin hue.

This is not that dissimilar from the Chinese idea of stressful events impacting in different areas on the face as you age. Instead of stress, it is sunbathing, being active outdoors, using sun beds etc. and from the severity of the aging features, you can get an idea of how much of their life was spent in the sun.

2. SMOKING

The number of packs you smoke a day and for how long directly correlates to the severity of your aging features[13]. There is even such a thing as a 'smoker's face' which is thin and bony with heavy wrinkles, and a greyish hue to the skin[14]. This is thought to happen as smoking damages tissues, reduces blood flow, and prevents nutrients and oxygen from reaching the skin.

3. DIET

The old adage 'you are what you eat' rings true with your face. One of the most obvious connections with diet and your face is the problem of acne vulgaris. Study upon study has linked the consumption of dairy products with the manifestation of acne spots[15]. It is however blamed on anything from a high glycaemic load diet to processed cheese and a high-fat diet. To anyone with even a passing knowledge of Oriental medicine, this connection would seem blindingly obvious and caused by heat disorders in the stomach, but medical studies have yet to join the dots properly.

A diet consisting mainly of processed, sugary foods as is so common nowadays can directly contribute to puffiness under your eyes which is quite literally an accumulation of fluids. Your stomach is so overwhelmed that your digestion can no longer adequately process fluids and starts storing it in the form of fat.

Your skin will also feel tighter as the collagen fibres which are being starved of nutrients, lose their flexibility.

Alcohol can directly cause a flushed complexion and a red nose, and too much can trigger a bout of Rosacea (rose-ay-sha), which features dilated blood vessels and redness on your nose and cheeks. It also dehydrates your skin and hair making it more likely that wrinkles and lines will deepen.

4. EXERCISE

The amount of exercise you do on a regular basis has a noticeable effect on your skin. Researchers in Canada have found that even in old age, regular jogging or cycling for 30 minutes twice a week can dramatically soften the outer layer of skin and create more elasticity in the dermis underneath[16]. If, however, you do not do regular exercise, you are much more likely to develop saggy, loose skin in your neck and jowls and your forehead and eye area can look fatter[17].

5. LACK OF SLEEP

The skin needs sleep. If you do not rest enough, it cannot regenerate properly and your face will start to show signs of this very quickly. One study looked at what happens to 30 women's faces when a normal 8-hour sleep pattern is reduced to 6 hours over a 5-day period. The results were that on average, lines and wrinkles increased in visibility by 45%, spots increased by 13%, red areas increased by 8% and brown spots increased by 11%[18]. If this sleep pattern were to continue, it is logical to presume that these temporary facial features would develop into more permanent ones.

Without at least acknowledging that these factors have a bearing on the state of your skin, any skin treatment plan that you do follow will be limited either in duration or in its long-term effects.

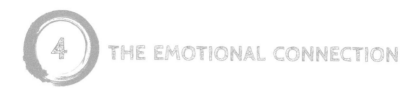

4 THE EMOTIONAL CONNECTION

THE MARCH OF LIFE

When many people start to notice signs of ageing in themselves, their focus is on the wrinkles, the creases and the sagging but what they are often feeling is an awareness of their own mortality. For some this represents a great fear and this emotion is transferred to a preoccupation with the state of their skin. Lines and wrinkles are a reminder that the march of life has no rest and that they are perhaps further along that path than they feel comfortable with.

YOUR FACE

It is probably obvious that if you experience strong emotions over a prolonged period or at a very deep level that the muscles involved may be used far more than others in the face. Over time, this repetition which showed on the skin as dynamic lines which came and went with each expression, is now replaced with static lines which exist whether or not you are making a facial expression or not.

THE FIVE ELEMENTS

One of the reasons Gua sha is effective is because it is based on ideas which encompass key human emotions and their effect on the body and face. You may be aware of a whole host of emotions that you go through on a daily basis but the ancient Chinese narrowed these down to a set of clinically useful emotions each with a different effect on your body and skin.

These emotions are grouped according to the five elements: Metal, Earth, Fire, Water and Wood. There is nothing mystical or new age about these elements. They were just a clever way for the ancient Chinese to express how the body functions in its natural environment. We now have other words and concepts to explain this, but the elements still serve as a simple and elegant way of organising ideas and they also can be represented by colours. You will notice that these colours feature throughout the book. Apart from the obvious aesthetic benefit of making it all look nice, the usefulness of this is that the colour itself can give you a clue about an organ, a channel, an element or emotion.

EMOTIONS OF METAL

KEY EMOTIONS

Grief, sadness, longing and detachment

KEY MUSCLES

Depressor anguli oris, orbicularis oculi, corrugator and depressor supercilii

DIRECT EFFECT ON FACE

○ The depressor anguli oris muscle (I) pulls your lip corners in a downward direction and is the main muscle associated with showing sadness and grief in the face. You just have to hold a mirror in front of your face and pull a 'sad' face. Watch your mouth and how the sides bend down (see image 3).

○ Try raising your cheeks at the same time. This is the orbicularis oculi muscle (C) pulling your cheeks up and it is often used together with the procerus (B), corrugator supercilii (D) and depressor supercilii muscles (E) to pull your eyebrows in and create a frown, or sometimes the frontalis muscle (A) to raise them up.

○ Common facial features generated by these emotions can be crow's feet next to your eyes, worry lines on your forehead, smile lines between your nose and the corners of your mouth and marionette lines from your mouth to your chin.

INDIRECT EFFECT ON FACE

These emotions are thought to affect two internal organs more than any others, your Lungs and Large intestines (these are the two organs of the Metal element).

○ According to the ancient Chinese, your lung is the organ most closely related to the strength and vitality of the skin. This is easy to see if you note the typical facial skin condition of a long-term smoker. It normally lacks moisture and often shows premature signs of ageing like crow's feet and the vertical lines around the mouth appropriately known as 'smoker's lines'. This is the result of a chronically weakened lung which is unable to disperse fluids in the body and nourish and moisturise the skin.

○ It is only recently that conventional medicine research is confirming this close relationship with the skin and the lungs. For example, the recognition of what is known as the 'atopic march' whereby the inflammatory response to atopic dermatitis is thought to cause asthma[19] or a recent study spanning 30 years which found that psoriasis sufferers are at a greater risk of developing chronic obstructive pulmonary disease than the general population[20].

○ This link with your lungs means that unresolved Metal will weaken the vitality of the skin as the repetition of muscle movement means that these muscles and the skin connected require nutrients, moisture and cellular energy far more than those which are less used. The irony is that they will actually receive less because the required amount is just not available. This means that there is more potential for developing static facial features such as lines and wrinkles.

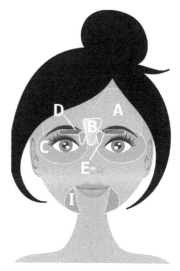

Image 3: Muscles of Metal/Earth

EMOTIONS OF EARTH

KEY EMOTIONS
Worry, pensiveness and over-thinking

KEY MUSCLES
Frontalis, corrugator supercilii and depressor supercilii muscles

DIRECT EFFECT ON FACE
(See image 3)

When you worry these are the actions of the facial muscles:

○ When you raise your forehead, the frontalis muscle (A) is lifting it up creating horizontal lines which span across your forehead.
○ This is combined with the corrugator supercilii (D) and

23

depressor supercilii muscles (E) pulling the eyebrows inwards and forming more lines vertically. This is the classic frowning expression.

- Possible static facial features generated by these emotions are worry lines and frown lines.

INDIRECT EFFECT ON FACE

- Studies have been published which look at how asking people to actively frown can negatively affect how they see the world and the physical act of frowning actually can cause a reduction in feelings of happiness and tolerance[21].
- Worry and over-thinking are thought to affect the two Earth organs, the Stomach and Spleen/Pancreas, both of which are heavily connected to your digestion. Too much thinking can therefore weaken digestion by interrupting the delicate system of how your stomach processes food. A weakening of your stomach also has implications directly for your forehead.
- Another very smart idea from the ancient Chinese was to map out the skin into zones of influence. This means that any area of skin can be directly linked to organs in your body and how well they may be functioning. The concept is called 'Cutaneous regions' and was featured in my first Gua sha book about your body and health. According to this theory, your stomach and intestines are most associated with the state of the skin on your face. This means that if your digestion has weakened, which is very possible if you are prone to worry and over-thinking or perhaps study for long hours, then you will often see changes in colour and texture of your skin.
- The effect on the face is compounded by the fact that one of the main functions of your Spleen/Pancreas in Oriental medicine is to ensure the transport of nutrients to your muscles and if not functioning well can help to cause muscle weakness and atrophy.

EMOTIONS OF FIRE

KEY EMOTIONS

Happiness, over-excitement, lack of self-acceptance, depression and self-loathing

KEY MUSCLES

Zygomaticus major, orbicularis oculi, nasalis, levator labii superioris alaeque nasi

DIRECT EFFECT ON FACE

(See image 4)

○ For joy and happiness, the zygomaticus major muscle (J) pulls the corner of your lips outwards towards your ears.

○ This is often accompanied by the orbicularis oculi muscle (C) lifting up your cheeks and scrunching up your eyes.

○ The nasalis (G) and levator labii alaeque nasi (H) muscles also contract, slightly scrunching your nose.

○ Try this in front of the mirror and you will see that you have the features of a classic happy, laughing face.

○ For the opposite feelings of depression and self-loathing, the expression and the effects on the face and body is very much like the one detailed in Metal with the depressor anguli oris (I) pulling the sides of your lips down. Ironically, whether happy or sad, smile lines are one of the key features of Fire emotions.

○ Possible static facial features generated by these emotions are smile lines between your nose and the corners of your mouth, crow's feet at the sides of your eyes and bunny lines at the side of your nose.

INDIRECT EFFECT ON FACE

○ Emotions of joy or the lack of it are connected to the Fire group of organs, the most prominent of which is your Heart. Of all the organs in the body, your heart is the most important and for this reason it was named the Emperor organ by the ancient Chinese.

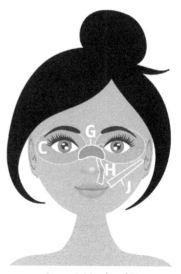

Image 4: Muscles of Fire

It is the pump which circulates nutrition-rich blood through the vascular system and ensures that the rest of your organs, muscles and tissues are well-serviced but it also represents something on a deeper emotional level. According to the classic Oriental medicine text from 240 BCE, The Yellow Emperor's Classic of Medicine, it is the very radiance of the spirit which stems from the heart.

○ If we say that someone is looking radiant, we are referring to their face and often something that is hard to define but clearly present. It is similar to pregnant women who are sometimes told that they are 'glowing' as hormone changes enhance the look of their facial skin. A healthy heart organ can affect this difficult-to-define glow or radiance of what the Chinese called your inner spirit or 'Shen'. And of course if your heart organ has become weak, the opposite is true.

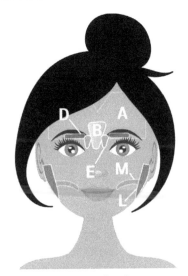

Image 5: Muscles of Water

EMOTIONS OF WATER

KEY EMOTIONS
Fear, isolation and insecurity

KEY MUSCLES
Frontalis, procerus, depressor supercilii and corrugator supercilii

DIRECT EFFECT ON FACE

Fear is usually shown when the lower part of your face is widened and pulled down (see image 5):

○ The frontalis (A) muscle lifts your eyebrows upwards.

○ The procerus (B), depressor supercilii (E) and corrugator supercilii muscles (D) bring your eyebrows together to form a frown.

○ The levator palpebrae superioris muscle (a very thin triangular muscle above your eye ball) simultaneously lifts your upper eyelids.

○ The risorius muscle (M) stretches your lips.

○ The masseter muscle (L) drops your jaw downwards.

○ Possible static facial features generated by these emotions are worry lines on your forehead and frown lines between your eyebrows.

INDIRECT EFFECT ON FACE

○ The two Water organs are the Kidneys and Bladder and it is here that the ancient Chinese believed to be the seat of courage and willpower. When weak these strong character traits turn to fear which then compounds the weakness further. As the kidneys are thought to control the growth and development of bones and nourish the marrow within them, the skin can become pale as the lack of red and white blood cells within the marrow can lead to anaemia and immune deficiency.

○ Dark circles can develop below your eyes when your kidneys are weak and exhausted. When your body is tired, it over-produces a chemical

called cortisol to energise the body. A side effect of this is that the volume of the blood in your body increases and the blood vessels enlarge. This change in blood flow can easily be seen under your eyes as the skin is particularly thin and can often be pale.

EMOTIONS OF WOOD

KEY EMOTIONS
Anger, resentment, frustration, timidity, shyness

KEY MUSCLES
Orbicularis oculi and orbicularis oris, procerus, depressor supercilii and corrugator supercilii

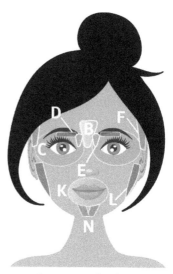

Image 6: Muscles of Wood

With anger the following muscular actions occur (see image 6):

- The orbicularis oculi muscle (C) contracts and tightens your eyes.
- The orbicularis oris muscle (K) and the mentalis muscle (N) tighten your lips.
- The three brow lowerers, the procerus (B), depressor supercilii (E) and corrugator supercilii (D) muscles, pull you eyebrows down to create vertical lines in the skin between them.
- The upper eyelid area is lifted by the levator palpebrae superioris (above your eyeball) to create a stare.
- The masseter muscle (L) and temporalis muscle (F) clench the jaw tightly.
- Possible static facial features generated by these emotions are frown lines between your eyebrows, crow's feet at the sides of your eyes and smile lines between your nose and mouth.

- Anger is associated with the two Wood organs, the Liver and Gall bladder. A well-functioning liver helps your blood to flow smoothly and uniformly throughout the body and when it gets disrupted, so too does the flow. Our muscles, tendons and tissues depend on a constant supply of fresh oxygenated blood but if the liver becomes chronically under-functioning which in Oriental medicine terms is rather like the control centre for the subway system, those muscles, tensions and tissues in the face will become more malnourished and weak.
- While it is perfectly normal to feel these emotions, the issue comes when the emotion is unresolved and is internalised. It is very common to hold in your feelings of frustration and anger which of course do not stop the frustration and anger, but allows them to stew inside your body and start to affect muscle tension and how the blood flows around your body and face.

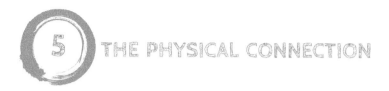

5 THE PHYSICAL CONNECTION

ANCIENT IDEAS

The connection between your facial muscles with the appearance of your skin is an obvious one, but you may not be aware of how much your face reflects not just what is happening in your face but what happening in your body. In order to understand this, let us look in more detail at ideas in Oriental medicine about how the two are connected. With this knowledge you can enhance the effectiveness of applying Gua sha for your face.

FACIAL COLOURS

When you look in the mirror you may have noticed that your (make-up free) complexion is not actually uniform in colour. The best way to see this is stand in front of a window to let natural light illuminate your face and hold up a hand mirror. Look for any colours, especially around your eyes and around your mouth. You may, like many people, notice shades of green, yellow, blue, red

and white. If you do, no need to panic or jump to any conclusions. All of these are common to be found in the face and each one has a specific meaning in Oriental medicine connected with the state of your body. When taken alone, these colours do not have much diagnostic value and have to be seen in the context of other signs and symptoms. You can find the following colours anywhere but image 7 shows the common sites:

RED Traditionally this is connected to an imbalance in the Fire element or too much heat. It is often connected to excess stimulation and can manifest with red cheeks.

GREEN You may see a green hue often around your mouth or around your eyes. This suggests an imbalance in Wood. It is often connected with anger, irritability and frustration, although strong feelings like hate may produce a greenish colour on the cheeks. Green is also often

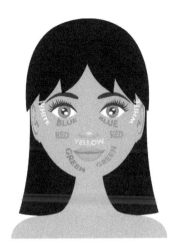

Image 7: Colours in your face

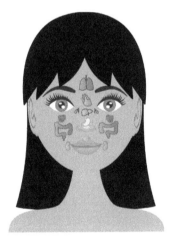

Image 8: Organs in your face

connected to menstrual problems, stress, and frustration.

YELLOW suggests an imbalance in Earth and is often connected to digestive problems and the retention of liquid in your body. It is also connected to overthinking and worrying. It is commonly seen around your mouth.

WHITE You may see white next to your eyes which can mean an imbalance in Metal or that cold is affecting your body. You might often be sad or depressed.

BLUE/PURPLE You may see blue or purple under your eyes which suggests an imbalance in Water. If long-term, it suggests that your lifestyle is weakening your body on a chronic level.

ORGANS IN FACE

Image 8 shows another traditional representation of how your body can appear in your face. This is less about colour and more about positioning. Designated areas of the face correspond to organs in your body with your lungs between your eyebrows and your heart, liver and gall bladder, and stomach and spleen down the nose. Your small intestines, large intestines and kidneys are in a line under your eyes, and your bladder above your mouth. Like the colours, these indications have limited diagnostic value when not seen in context, but they provide yet another example of how your face can offer up a treasure trove of information if you know where to look.

THE PRIMARY CHANNELS

Pick up virtually any book or click on any link about Oriental medicine and you will be sure to come across images with colourful lines all over the body. These are detailing the 12 primary channels (see images 9 and 10) which make up a neurovascular system which distributes nutrients, oxygen and vital substances all over your body in a subway-map like formation. The whole network runs through your body's connective tissue which, as its name suggests, connects, supports and anchors all the separate pieces of our bodies.

GUA SHA ALONG LINES

Just like the subway system, each of the coloured lines represents a distinct channel or vessel and has different origins and destinations around the body. The dots along these lines represent points or nodes which

if manipulated appropriately can cause a physiological reaction and increase circulation along this channel and so affect muscles and organs connected to it. Research has shown that microcirculation and the body's transference of blood from vessels to the capillary bed in the tissues (known as blood perfusion volume) shows a distinct increase if applying Gua sha directly along a channel and at the points which lie along it[22].

For this reason the channel system is very important to keep in mind when doing Gua sha.

It should not prove to be too taxing in working out these channels as most of the lines have the same names as organs in the body and usually have a direct physical connection with those organs i.e. they often pass through them. They are traditionally paired together with the name of one of the 5 elements in order to help reach a deeper meaning of how they work together.

METAL CHANNELS (GREY)

- ○ Lung (LU): from your chest to your thumb
- ○ Large Intestine (LI): from your thumb to your nose

EARTH CHANNELS (YELLOW)

- ○ Stomach (ST) – from your head to your second toe

31

FACIAL GUA SHA

- Spleen (SP) – from your big toe to your chest

FIRE CHANNELS (RED)

- Heart (HT) – from your armpit to your little finger
- Small Intestine (SI) – from your little finger to ear
- Pericardium (PC) – from your chest to middle finger
- Triple burner (TB) – from your ring finger to your temple

WATER CHANNELS (BLUE)

- Kidney (KD) – from your sole to the front of your chest
- Bladder (BL) – from your eye to little toe via your back

WOOD CHANNELS (GREEN)

- Gall bladder (GB) – from your eye to 4th toe
- Liver (LV) – from your big toe to your chest

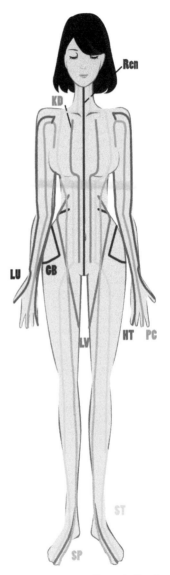

Image 9: Primary Channels (front)

32

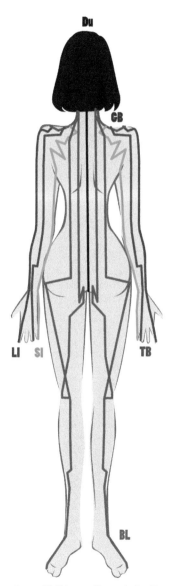

Image 10: Primary Channels (back)

EXTRA CHANNELS

These are not considered part of the 12 primary channels but are related and feature heavily in any treatment of the 12 primary channels.

- ⭕ Ren (brown) – from your genital area to your chin on the front of your body
- ⭕ Du (black) – from your top lip to below your bottom on the back of your body

FACE CHANNELS

Knowledge of this system is very useful when thinking about treatments on your face. This is because one of each pair of channels in the body runs directly over the facial area. These are known as the Yang channels. The ones that stop or start in the body rather than the head are called the Yin channels.

As an extension of the body channels, image 11 show the same channels in more detail over the neck and facial area.

- ⭕ Ren - on the centre-line above your lips.
- ⭕ Du - on the centre-line below your lips.
- ⭕ Large intestine (LI) - ends at the side of your nostril.
- ⭕ Gall bladder (GB) - passes

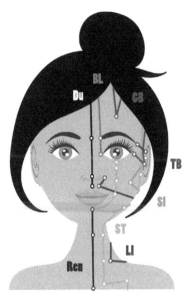

Image 11: Primary Channels (face)

over the side of your head to your eye.

○ Stomach (ST) - branches into two lines across your face

○ Triple burner (TB) - around your ear and to your eyebrow.

○ Small intestine (SI) - across your cheek to your ear.

○ Bladder (BL) - over the top of your head.

As can be seen in these images, your face is connected to your body through this intricate network. Remember that these are not imaginary energetic channels flowing through your body but demonstrable planes in the connective tissue. One of the

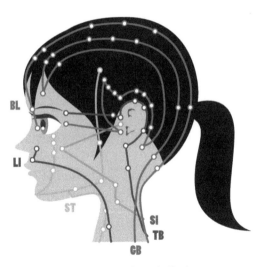

Image 12: Primary Channels (face)

clearest ways of seeing this is to look at how these channels work in tandem with another layer known as the Tendino-muscular channels. And to explore this, we need to start with the skin.

SKIN LAYERS

If you analyse the skin, you will note that rather than being one unified piece sitting between your innards and the outside world, there are layer upon layer of tissue each with its own distinct function (see image 13).

1. The epidermis is the outer most layer and protects the body by making new skin cells and producing melanin.
2. The dermis is sandwiched underneath with the blood vessels, sweat glands, hair roots and nerve endings.
3. Below this is the subcutaneous fat which contains connective tissue, provides padding and helps control the body temperature.

Each of these layers can be sub-divided into further layers with further functions and if we look at the subcutaneous fat of the face, we can find something called the superficial muscular aponeurotic system (SMAS) which is sandwiched between the deep and superficial facial fat.

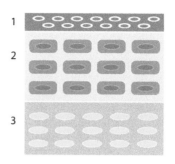

Image 13: Skin layers

SMAS

This is often referred to in facial lifting surgeries and it is thought to be an extensive fibromuscular layer which interconnects the expressive muscles of your face. As the SMAS distributes the contractions of these facial muscles to the skin, any changes to it will have an impact on the appearance of your skin. The SMAS therefore acts as a continuous membranous link from muscle to muscle, tendon to tendon and tissue to tissue in your face. This was first suggested in scientific circles by two researchers in 1976 but actually this type of linkage was described in Chapter 13 of the Spiritual Pivot, part of the Yellow Emperor's Inner Classic, a book written in China in the second century CE. This was called the theory of the Jingjin which can loosely be translated as the Tendino-muscular channels.

TENDINO-MUSCULAR LAYER

If we looked at the channel system like we did the skin, we would see that below the skin and above the principal channels we looked at earlier, are the Tendino-muscular (TM) channels which connect the muscles, tendons and ligaments and tissues, joints and skin (see images 14 and 15).

MUSCLE NETWORK

To help you avoid any confusion, these TM channels mainly follow a very similar route over the body as the principal channels. The colours in the illustration are also the same: Gall bladder is green, Stomach is yellow, Bladder is blue, Large intestine is dark grey, Small intestine is red and Triple burner is purple. The main difference is that rather than lines snaking over the body, these channels flow through the connective tissue network in a thick band through major muscle groups. So if we followed the TM channels, we would be going from whole muscle to whole muscle up or down along the body, roughly in line with the trajectory of the primary channels.

STOMACH TM CHANNEL

Take the Stomach TM channel (ST) as an example. Almost all the muscles in your face below your eye level are considered part of the Stomach TM channel. It continues downwards at the front of your neck with the stemohyoid and stemothyroid muscles. It then jumps down to the rectus abdominus and the psoas and iliacus muscles behind. It then leads on to your big thigh frontal muscles – the vastus lateralis, vastus intermedius and rectus femoris – then the tibialis anterior on your lower leg and the extensor digitorum longus and extensor hallusis brevis at your ankle and foot. If we were to superimpose the Stomach primary channel onto this muscular picture, you would see that the line passes perfectly through each of these muscle area.

IMPORTANCE OF TM LAYER

The importance of these TM channels in terms of the face is that they provide an external source of cell energy, nutrients and oxygen for the muscles, tendons and ligaments and help control reflexive muscle actions in your body, much like the SMAS as described earlier. This means that when you raise your

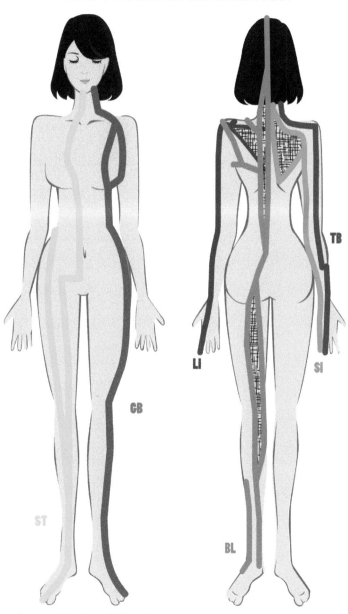

Image 14: TM Channels (front)   Image 15: TM Channels (back)

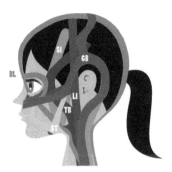

Image 16: TM Channels (head)

eyebrows instinctively to express surprise, the muscles are drawing on this fibromuscular source in order to move effectively. It also can mean that one of the signs of a problem of blood flow in these channels is when muscles become lax and lose their elasticity.

COMBINING THE CHANNELS

For Gua sha treatments to be more effective, this knowledge of the trajectories of the channels (both primary and TM) can be combined, so that instead of local treatment to the facial muscles, you can treat the channel further down the body in order to make changes to your face.

For example, you may notice that the dark green line of the Gall Bladder (GB) primary channel runs down the forehead, stops and then goes up again making a V-shape. At the apex of the V is a point which, when stimulated,

affects the forehead and eye area. In order to treat the forehead, you might stimulate this Gall bladder point directly by scraping in this area. What you can also do, however, is to follow the Gall bladder channel as it runs down your body and scrape along muscle areas. You might also Gua sha its paired Wood channel, the Liver, or any other channels which can affect the Gall Bladder channel such as the Heart or Triple burner channels. All of these can have an effect on the Gall bladder channel and specifically on the side of the head and forehead.

This is the theory behind the Gua sha sequences that you will be following in the treatment section of the book.

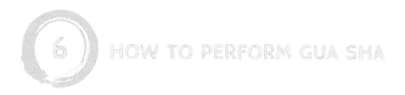

6 HOW TO PERFORM GUA SHA

EQUIPMENT

Facial Gua sha does not need any specialized tools in order to work. You can buy tools with a whole range of shapes and materials from specialist shops or on the internet but you can also use your fingers or a Chinese soup spoon and still get very similar benefits from Gua sha. In our clinic we have just about every shape, size and material of Gua sha tool but in our experience, it is not the tool which you should fixate about but how to use it effectively.

TOOL-FREE SCRAPING

The simplest and quickest way to use Gua sha on your face is to use your hands, instead of a tool.

In order to do this you need to get your hand shape correct.

1. Create a fist and tuck your thumb under your index finger. Use the flat surface of the middle metatarsal bone of the index finger for the stroking.

The main joint of the index finger can also be used to press points (see image 17).

2. For areas in which this flat fist shape cannot reach, you can adjust your index finger so that it lifts up (see image 18).

HAND SCRAPING TECHNIQUE

Using the flat part of the middle section of the index finger, drag your hands across the skin as you would with a Gua sha tool. Follow the same general procedures of tool Gua sha and ensure that the angle of the middle section of the index finger is at 90 degrees to the skin.

Treat only one side at a time – usually the left side with your left hand and the right side with your right hand but the opposite is fine. Keep a constant pressure and speed so that it is firm but comfortable.

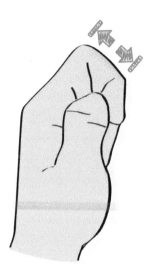

Image 17: Scraping hand shape

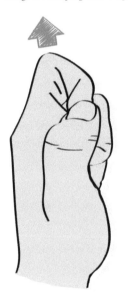

Image 18: Scraping finger shape

SCRAPING WITH A TOOL

Any Gua sha tool can be used for facial Gua sha but a smaller tool is more preferable for the face area - it is easier to manipulate and control. A tool which has a concave dent in it like some of the shaped resin ones that you can see in many of the illustrations in this book has the additional benefit of following the edge of the jaw line (one of the techniques for a double chin for example). Whichever tool you use, be aware of its shape and ensure that there is a longer edge represented in image 19 by the rectangle and a shorter rounded edge, shown by the circle.

Remember that while a specially made Gua sha tool is great and if you can get hold of one, I thoroughly recommend it, but you do not need to buy anything special to do facial Gua sha. A Chinese soup spoon is perfectly adequate for Gua sha treatment of the face. The benefits of a Chinese soup spoon (see image 20) are that they are easily purchased, inexpensive and made of porcelain which makes them easy to clean and cheap to replace (when you inevitably drop it).

PRESSURE

When treating the body, a varying amount of pressure is needed depending on the body part. If it is an area with a large thick muscle such as the mid back, pressure can be increased with each stroke of the Gua sha tool. The face however does not require the same pressure. In fact, in some areas the skin is very thin and can easily be damaged with the tool. It is important therefore to be consistent with the amount of pressure applied as you move the tool across your face and to press relatively lightly. Press just enough to stretch the skin and no more. The last thing most people want on their face is the red dots of petechiae to appear.

LUBRICANT

FOR YOUR FACE

If you just scrape a Gua sha tool across your face, the friction between your skin and the tool may not be that pleasant an experience. You therefore need some form of lubrication to provide a barrier so that the tool glides over rather than digs in the skin.

Small quantities of facial oils or creams are ideal as lubrication. Simple moisturizing cream is perfectly sufficient. You do not need to spend a lot of money on lubri-

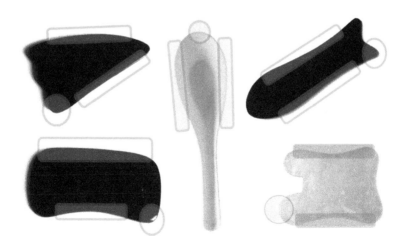

Image 19: Gua sha tools

41

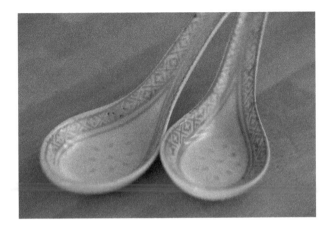

Image 20: Soup spoon

cant if you do not wish to - soap and water are great. You just need to ensure that the lubricant is not one which is quickly absorbed into the skin as it would then lose its lubricating effect. Oils that you might use for body Gua sha will probably not be appropriate for your face but there are a huge variety of oils and creams that can be used to facilitate and enhance the treatment in term of skin care. As far as which is the best depends on what kind of skin you have.

In Oriental medicine, for example, avocado-based products are thought to strengthen the consistency of your blood and lubricate your lungs and intestines. When applied to the skin in the form of avocado-based oil it has a similar lubricating and strengthening quality and is thought to improve skin hydration and elasticity.

Sesame-based oils are another great lubricating oil. Inside the body it is used to lubricate the intestines and so help constipation, and on the skin to combat dry and cracked areas.

Evening primrose is believed to regulate fluids in the body. It is well-known for its high concentration of a fatty acid called gamma-linolenic acid which is thought to regulate cellular functions to have anti-inflammatory properties.

The choice of oils and creams is wide and varied and people often have a preference, so choose the most appropriate for your skin. But do not get too hung up about the lubrication. It is the Gua sha that makes the changes not so much your choice of oils or creams.

FOR YOUR BODY

For the Gua sha treatments on the rest of your body where your skin is usually less delicate, you can use anything from blended massage oils or vegetable oils you can find in the kitchen to Vapour rub or Vaseline. If you prefer, you can also scrape over light clothing without the need for lubrication. If you have any skin issues of course you need to take that into account.

GUA SHA TECHNIQUES

There are important stroking techniques which are used frequently in facial Gua sha which are quite distinct from those used in other parts of the body. These techniques are gentler and are about supporting and strengthening the face and body.

With any aesthetic treatment to the face great care should be taken not to mark the skin. The idea is to be firm but very light and if any marks were to appear, reassess what you are doing immediately.

The main techniques are the following:

A. SWEEP

○ Use the side of the Gua sha tool (see the tool section for more details) but each stroke is a continual unbroken movement from beginning to end. It is a flowing action much like cleaning the windows with a long rubber blade, ironing the crease out of a sheet or the movement of a paint brush along the canvas (see image 21).

○ Slightly press on the tool as you sweep but just deep enough to nudge the muscle and tissue.

○ Steady contact between the tool and the skin is maintained the whole time.

○ The technique should leave the skin slightly and temporarily flushed but should not leave any redness or skin discolouration.

B. MOVING CIRCLE

○ Use the rounded corner of the tool and applying light pressure only, slowly move forwards using a circular motion (see image 22).

○ Steady contact between the tool and the skin is maintained the whole time.

○ This should result in nothing more than slightly flushed skin with no redness.

C. STATIC CIRCLE

○ Static circle is a fixed circular movement at one point using the corner of the tool. It is used with only a little pressure and in more sensitive areas such as the temples and near the eyes (see image 23).

○ The tool touches the skin at one fixed point and the circle movement is from your arm and wrist and in the tissue and muscle underneath not on the skin surface.

D. WIDE STROKE

○ Use the side part of the Gua sha tool to press and stroke (at the same time) with the tool. Each stroke should be measured, firm and have consistent pressure (see image 24).

○ Wide stroke has shorter, stronger strokes than the sweep technique.

○ This technique is used over the head and on the body and can generate 'sha' on the skin.

E. NARROW STROKE

○ This technique is similar to wide stroke. The difference is that you use the rounded end of the tool to stroke instead of the longer side, which means that the surface area of the skin treated is much narrower and the effect is therefore more focused and stronger (see image 25).

○ This technique is used on the body and like wide stroke can generate 'sha'.

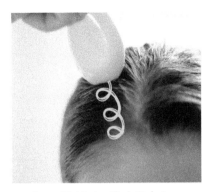

Image 22: Moving Circle Technique

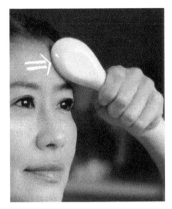

Image 21: Sweep Technique

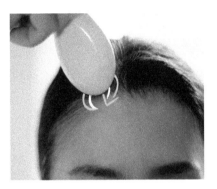

Image 23: Static Circle Technique

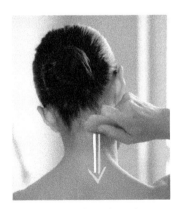

Image 24: Wide Stroke Technique

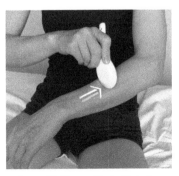

Image 25: Narrow Stroke Technique

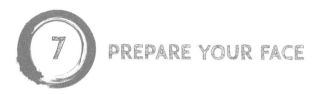

7 PREPARE YOUR FACE

TONE YOUR FACE

CAUTION

It may seem obvious but do not perform Gua sha on your eyes, lips, tongue, nostrils or near your ear canal, as the stroking may damage these more sensitive areas of skin.

If you have pimples, spots, or any raised skin features on your skin, do not scrape over them. If it is a small area, you can cover it with your finger of your other hand as you scrape or sweep around it. For larger affected areas, they are best avoided. Instead scrape over areas of your body which treat that area.

LOOSENING SEQUENCE

Just like physical exercise, before treating and toning the facial muscles, tissues and their related areas, you should warm them up. This can be done with the following loosening sequence which is designed to loosen the mus-cles in the facial and head area. Each time you treat, first loosen the muscles with these gentle exercises and therefore reduce the likelihood of Gua sha treatment producing unwanted petechiae or 'sha' marks on your skin.

A. LOOSEN YOUR HEAD

Firstly, indirectly relax your facial muscles by loosening your head. This is actually a technique which works on many levels.

○ It ensures that the large muscle and tissue groups like the galea aponeurotica (the membrane over the top of your head), the occipitalis (at the back of the head), the temporalis, the temporoparietetalis and the auricularis (which are all at the side of your head) become less tense which will indirectly loosen the face.

○ As each of these muscle and tissue groups correspond to TM channels (the Bladder, Gall bladder, Triple burner and Small intestine respectively) it also means that it is not only the localised muscle areas which are being loosened but further along these muscle channels (for more on the TM channels see Chapter 5).

○ It is also represents direct stimulation of the Du, Gall bladder, Bladder and Triple burner primary channels which run over the head area. So while it appears you are just dragging a blunt object over the top of the skin, you are actually doing something far more meaningful and profound to your health and wellbeing.

HEAD SEQUENCE

Note: This sequence is mostly within the hairline and no lubrication is needed for your head if you have hair. If not and for any parts which have lost their hair, lubricate as you would any part of the body.

1. Start with a static circle technique. Continue for about 5 seconds at each of the three points at the frontal hairline: one on the midline, one at the corner of the head, and one in between (see image 26).

2. Next, use a moving circle technique from the mid-point down to the front of your ear (see image 27). Repeat three times.

3. Continue the moving circle technique but this time from the top of your forehead backwards over your head (see image 28). Start near the centre line and circle back over your head towards your occiput. Then repeat twice more, each time moving the line closer to the side of your head.

4. Use a moving circle technique from the front of your ear, go around the top and then continue behind it (see image 29). Repeat three times.

5. From the back of your ear continue the movement down the side of the neck (see image 30). Change from a moving circle technique to a sweep technique as you stroke down the neck muscles. Repeat three times.

6. Use a static circle technique at the midpoint of the occiput at the back of the head for 5 seconds. Then static circle one point either side, about three finger widths away, for 5 seconds each. Ensure you are in the muscle below the bone and not on the skull (see image 31).

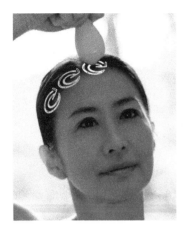

Image 26: Head Step 1

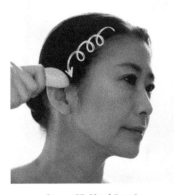

Image 27: Head Step 2

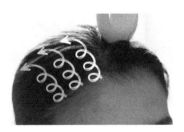

Image 28: Head Step 3

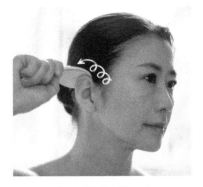

Image 29: Head Step 4

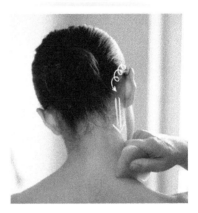

Image 30: Head Step 5

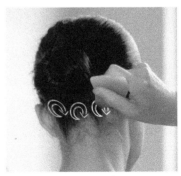

Image 31: Head Step 6

7. Repeat steps 1-5 on the other side of your head. And then repeat step 6.

B. LOOSEN YOUR FACE

Like your head, loosening your face is far more than just lightly circling a Gua sha tool over the surface of the skin. Your face is full of points, channels and muscle groups and this technique provides the initial local stimulation and relaxation before local Gua sha treatment.

FACE SEQUENCE

Spread a small amount of lubricant on your face smoothly, ensuring there is enough to lightly lubricate but not too much to make it slippery.

Repeat each part on the other side of your face.

1. Place the corner of the instrument at the midpoint in between your eyebrows. Then use a moving circle technique up your forehead to just below your natural hairline. Repeat this line a second time. Move a finger width closer to the temple and repeat this circular movement up the forehead. Each line should go up parallel to the previous one until the edge of the forehead. And each circular line should be repeated three to four times. It is very important that the pressure is light and the movement is firm but gentle (see image 32).

2. Start in between your eyebrows and circle (moving) outwards along your eyebrow to the end. Repeat again above the eyebrow (see image 33). Repeat three times.

3. Static circle at your temple area - press lightly with the corner of the tool while making a circular movement. Continue this for 10 seconds (see image 33).

4. Start at the inside corner of your eye and circle (moving) around your lower eye socket. Finish at the temple (see image 34).

5. Start at the side of your nose, around half way down and follow the cheek bone circling (moving) around to the temple (see image 34).

6. Start at corner of your lips and circle (moving) out and upwards to the temple (see image 34).

7. From the midpoint of your chin, circle (moving) outwards and upwards to the temple (see

image 34). Repeat steps 4-7 three times.

8. Return to the midpoint of your chin but go lower, just below the jaw bone and follow it around until below the ear (see image 35). Repeat three times.

9. Circle from below the nasolabial groove to the sides of your nostrils. Circle (moving) upwards and at the bridge of the nose, follow the eye socket around again and finish at the temples (see image 36). Repeat three times.

10. Repeat steps 1-9 on the other side of your face.

The Head and Face loosening sequences are designed to be done together as a set of movements to help relax all of the important muscle groups and channels over the head and face. Once relaxed, they are then ready for the treatment phase.

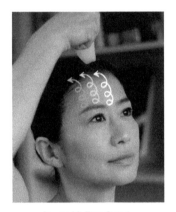

Image 32: Face Step 1

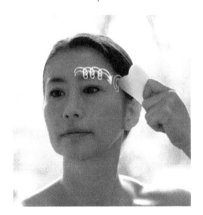

Image 33:
Face Steps 2 & 3

Image 34:
Face Steps 4,5,6 and 7

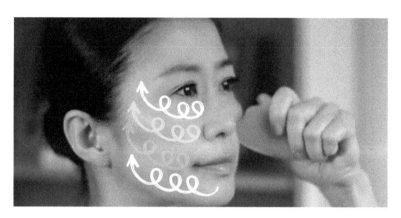

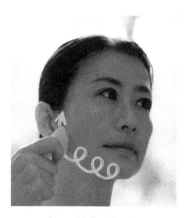

Image 35: Face Step 8

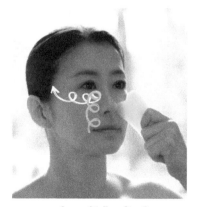

Image 36: Face Step 9

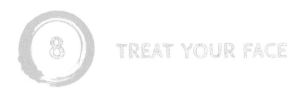

8 TREAT YOUR FACE

1. FOREHEAD AREA

COMMON AGING FEATURES

Worry lines, frown lines and brow ptosis

MUSCLES AND TISSUES

You may have noticed that the skin of your forehead is much thicker than that of your face. It is made up of multiple layers of skin, subcutaneous/loose connective tissue and sweat glands. It also contains several muscles which control your facial expression, known as 'mimetic' muscles. In fact the forehead area can be divided into three distinct regions each of which is relevant to treatment with Gua sha (see image 37).

REGION 1

The central part of the forehead contains the largest of the mimetic muscles, the frontalis (A), which is the frontal part of the thin epicranius muscle stretching all the way over your head to below the occiput. It covers most of the forehead area and splits neatly into two distinct halves, either side of the forehead. The skin in this area does not have much elasticity and is closely fixed to the muscle (See image 38).

REGION 2

The eyebrow area is dominated by the brow depressors which are made up of the following:

○ The procerus muscle (B) is a triangular shaped muscle which starts on the fascia of your nasal bone and rises up to insert into the skin between your eyebrows.
○ Under both eyebrows are the corrugator supercilii muscles (D) which start at the top of the nose and pass under the eyebrows behind the orbicularis oculi muscle (C), and insert into the skin.
○ The depressor supercilii muscles (E) are small muscles

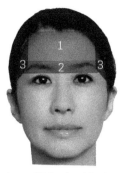

Image 37: Forehead Regions

which extend under your eyebrows and which work closely with the orbicularis oculi muscle (C).

○ These act together to pull the eyebrows inwards and downwards, forming vertical lines on the bridge of your nose and a frown in the forehead area.

REGION 3

The two lateral sides of your forehead lead into the temple area which rather than the convex frontalis muscle area, becomes more concave as the skin attaches to the temporalis fascia (F).

The region of most interest in this forehead-focused section is Region 1 as the frontalis muscle is the main detractor in the upper part of the face. It helps you to lift your eyebrows and it is used

repeatedly during any conversation.

Over time the thickening and lengthening of this muscle can create chronic contraction and horizontal lines known as 'worry lines'.

CHANNELS AND POINTS

In order to understand this area in terms of Oriental medicine, we need to look at the channels that run through each area.

REGION 1

The Gall bladder (GB) and Bladder (BL) channels start at your face, go over the head and all the way down your back and legs to finish at your toes.

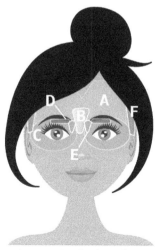

Image 38: Forehead Muscles

The Du channel starts below your coccyx bone underneath your bottom and comes straight up the spine, over the centre line of your head and stops above your mouth (see image 39).

Any local Gua sha treatment of the front part of your forehead area will affect these three channels. Likewise, if you treat these same channels further down your body, you can affect your forehead.

GB-14 (Yang White) is a point located two finger widths directly upwards from the centre point of the eyebrow (see image 40). It is located at the origin of the galea aponeurotica fibrous band which stretches over the top of the head. It has a strong influence on your eyes and eyelids as well as the forehead and is actually the meeting point of four primary channels. It is also the point of insertion of the motor nerve in the muscle fibres which means that stimulation here can reverberate across the muscle mass. As far as treatment of the forehead goes, this point is therefore essential.

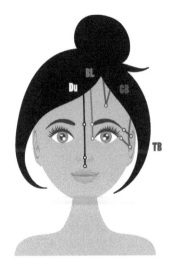

Image 39: Forehead Channels

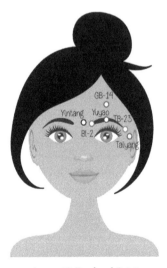

Image 40: Forehead Points

REGION 2

The same channels flow through this area with the addition of the Triple burner channel (TB). This channel starts at your ring finger and rises up over your arm, shoulder, neck and ear before finishing at your eyebrow. The last point is TB-23 (Silken Bamboo Hollow) which is at the site of the insertion of the frontalis muscle where it connects with the skin of eyebrows. The point affects the head, face, eyebrows and eyes and is located at the outer end of the eyebrows.

This area also contains many key points often used in treatment such as:

○ Yuyao (Fish Waist) is in the centre of the eyebrow and influences the eyes and relaxes tendons.

○ Yintang (Hall of Impression) is at the glabella and at the insertion of the motor nerve in the middle of the procerus muscle. It has influence over nasal congestion, headaches and calming your mind.

○ Bladder 2 (Gathered Bamboo) is directly above the corner of the eye at the start of the eyebrow. It influences the whole eyebrow area, eyes and headaches.

REGION 3

The Gall bladder channel (GB) starts and Triple burner channel (TB) finishes close to the corner of your eye (see image 39). Both channels run through the temple area and are connected to the outside of your arms (Triple burner) and the outside of your legs (Gallbladder).

Taiyang (Supreme Yang) lies in the temple at the level of your eyes. It affects the temple area, the face and eyes. It is one of the key danger areas in martial arts where direct contact is avoided.

FOREHEAD SEQUENCE

Gua sha for your forehead should include local face and head treatment combined with distal treatment on your arms and legs. The reason for these areas are as follows:

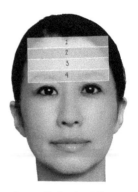

Image 41: Forehead Parts

○ Local treatment on your forehead area will affect the forehead muscles themselves and provide local stimulation of the three main channels and key points.

○ Treatment on your head will affect the epicranius muscle which stretches from your forehead over to the occiput bone at the bottom of your skull. The same three acupuncture channels also cover this whole area.

○ The arms and legs are to provide distal treatment to affect the three channels. Distal treatments are one of the corner stones to effective channel treatments in Oriental medicine.

ON YOUR FOREHEAD

Divide your forehead into four equal horizontal parts (see image 41).

1. Upper forehead to hairline: Start with your tool on the centre line of your upper forehead and sweep across the forehead to the temple area. This action should be smooth as if you were ironing bed sheets or stroking a pet. At the temple adjust the tool so that the whole side is in contact with the skin (like the position of the tool in wide stroke) and sweep up above the ear. The whole thing is one movement. The side of the tool gently pulls at the skin as it moves and makes full side contact with the temple area (see image 42).

2. Middle forehead: Repeat this slightly lower over the mid-forehead area (Region 1), into the temple (Region 2) and over your ear.

3. Lower forehead: Repeat this over the lower forehead (Region 1), into the temple (Region 2) and over your ear.
4. Eyebrows: From the midpoint between your eyebrows sweep across the eyebrows (Region 3) into the temple area (Region 2).

Repeat this sequence three to five times.

ON YOUR HEAD

5. As the frontalis muscle is directly connected to the galea aponeurotica membrane on your head, and whose origin is at the occipitalis at the back of the head, it should make perfect sense to wide stroke over your head towards the occiput. Always stroke towards the back of your head. Start at the top of your forehead and work backwards to the occiput with short firm strokes (see images 43 and 44). Repeat this several times but do not repeat the same area, each time moving down on either side.
6. At the occiput area, narrow stroke up and down along the occiput, where the neck meets the back of your skull. You can do this quickly at the speed of brushing your teeth (see image 45). In this way you are in

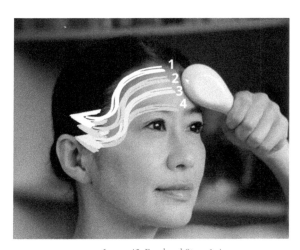

Image 42: Forehead Steps 1-4

effect treating the origin of the frontalis muscle. Do this for several repetitions.

ON YOUR BODY

7. Wide stroke upwards along the external oblique muscles at the side of your body (see image 46). These form part of the Gall Bladder TM channel group of muscles. Ensure you have enough lubricant to make the scraping comfortable if you scrape directly on your skin. Repeat several times.

ON YOUR ARMS

8. Wide stroke up (towards your body) along the Triple burner (TB) and Small intestine (SI) channels on the outside of your arm (see image 47) - for illustration purposes the Small intestine is shown on the inside. See images 48 and 49 for the TM muscle groups of these channels. Ensure you lubricate the area before scraping. Repeat several times.

9. Wide stroke down the Lung (LU) and Heart (HT) on the inside of your arm (see image 50). Stroke along the main muscle groups (see images 51 and 52) but avoid the bony parts of the elbow and wrist. Repeat several times.

ON YOUR LEGS

10. Wide stroke down (away from your body) the Bladder (BL) and Gall bladder (GB) channels on the outside of your leg (see image 53). The muscles which cover the Bladder TM channel can be seen in image 54 and the Gall Bladder TM channel in image 55. Make sure the area you scrape along is lubricated. Repeat several times.

11. Also wide stroke up the paired channels Kidney (KD) and Liver (LV) on the inside of your leg (see image 56). Be careful not to stroke directly on the tibia bone at the front of your lower leg nor over the bony parts of your knee. See images 57 and 58 for the Kidney and Liver TM muscle groups. Repeat several times.

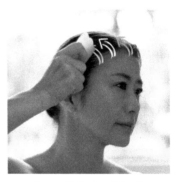

Image 43: Forehead Step 5

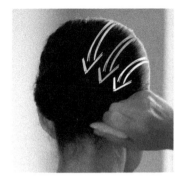

Image 44: Forehead Step 5

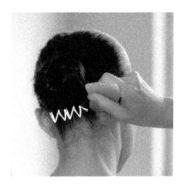

Image 45: Forehead Step 6

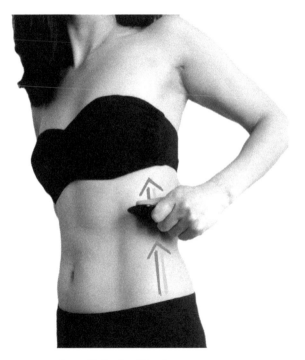

Image 46: Forehead Step 7

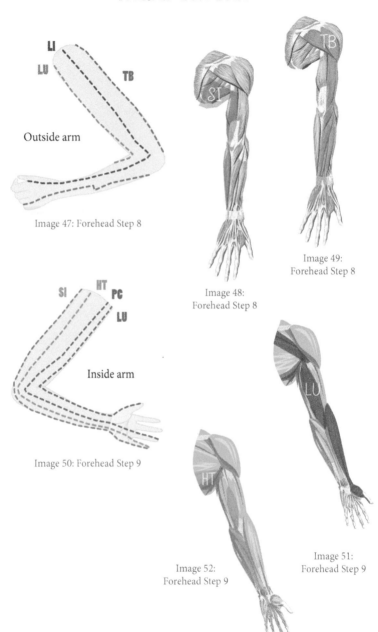

Image 47: Forehead Step 8

Outside arm

Image 48:
Forehead Step 8

Image 49:
Forehead Step 8

Inside arm

Image 50: Forehead Step 9

Image 52:
Forehead Step 9

Image 51:
Forehead Step 9

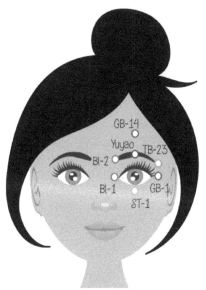

Image 61: Eye Points

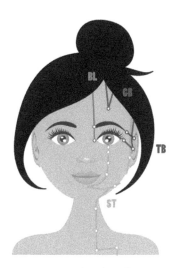

Image 60: Eye channels

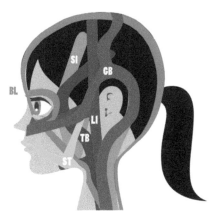

Image 62: Eye TM Channels

the orbicularis oculi (C) muscle (see images 59 and 61).

All of the face TM channels pass over this region (see image 62): Bladder (BL), Triple Burner (TB), Small intestine (SI) Stomach (ST) and Gall bladder (GB). Improving the circulation in these TM channels both locally and more distally, will have reverberations on the local tissue around your eyes.

BAGGY UPPER EYELIDS

The Gall bladder channel is traditionally connected to the upper eyelid and GB-14 (Yang White) which is actually above your eye on the forehead, is believed to have a strong influence on this area of your eyes (see image 61).

The Bladder channel starts at the inside corner of your eyes with BL-1 (Bright eyes) and then BL-2 (Gathered bamboo) at the start of your eyebrows. Both of these are indicated strongly to treat your eye lids (see image 61).

Across from BL-2 are Yuyao (Fish waist) in the middle of your eyebrow and TB-23 in the groove at the other end of the eyebrow. Both of these are directly above the upper eyelid (see image 61).

DARK RINGS

In terms of Oriental medicine, this is a good example of how the face reflects what is happening inside the body.

It is an area traditionally thought to be connected to the strength of your kidney function and the more distinct the colour, the weaker the core functions of the kidneys/adrenals usually are (which are connected to water metabolism, reproduction, bones and teeth, respiration and the storage of essential substances).

If, for example, you were to have too many late nights, you might have a temporary dark colour under the eyes to indicate that the balance in your kidneys has been disturbed. This has little connection to the day to day functioning of the kidney organ and with a good night's rest may then disappear as quickly as it came. If however you continue with an under-functioning kidney, these rings, known as periorbital dark circles, may make more frequent or permanent appearances.

This means that treatment via the Bladder channel, the paired organ with the Kidney, can both support your kidneys and influence your under-eye area, especially considering the fact that the Bladder TM channel (BL) runs directly through the tissue under your eyes (see image 62).

The Large intestine and Stomach TM channels also run in the area under the eyes and will be influential in improving circulation. The Stomach primary channel also begins at your eye socket directly below your eyeball with ST-1 (Container of tears) and cuts down through the under eye area (see images 60 and 61).

In order to make changes here, you really need to look at the state of your body in general and perhaps your lifestyle - more sleep, better stress management and an overhaul of your diet. It is useful to note also that as you age, your core vital substances reduce which is why these rings are often associated with aging.

BAGS UNDER EYES

In Oriental medicine, puffy or swollen eyes are a sign of excess fluids in the body but not just under the eye. These excess fluids are thought to accumulate in your body usually due to a weakness in your digestive organs and build up in the eye area partly due to the location of the Stomach channel which begins under the eyeball at ST-1 (see images 60 and 61). It is also connected to the

filter functioning of the Liver and Kidney.

It is therefore important that as well as treating the eye area locally, that key channels and points related to the accumulation of fluids and strengthening digestion are added in to the sequence.

As mentioned in the dark rings section, the Bladder (BL) and the Stomach (ST) TM channels converge in the orbicularis oculi muscle under your eyes and the Large intestine (LI) TM channel passes below your eye to bind at the side of your nose (see image 62). All three will help make changes in the under-eye area and can be treated locally and distally.

EYE SEQUENCE

ON YOUR FACE

1. Corner press Bl-2 which is at the start of your eyebrow, close to your nose. Divide your eyebrow into 3 equal parts and narrow stroke along your eyebrow in three strokes. At the end of your eyebrow sweep outwards towards your temple and at the temple, sweep up above the ear. The side of the tool gently pulls the skin in the crow's feet area as it comes off the eyebrow and makes full contact with the temple area. Repeat three to five times (see image 63).

2. Next repeat this but along the lower part of the eye socket instead. Press Bl-1 and then gently pass the corner of the eye and sweep around your eye socket under your eyes from the side of the nose. Follow the contour of the eye socket to your temple in one singular movement. At the temple slide up above ear again. Repeat three to five times (see image 63).

3. Move lower down the nose and repeat. Sweep from the side of the nose across to the temple. This time below the lower eye socket. At the temple slide up above ear again. Repeat three to five times (see image 63).

ON YOUR BACK

For dark rings under your eyes, add the following:

4. Wide stroke down your lower back on the large muscle groups either side of your spine (but not actually on the spine). Stroke down into your buttock area. Start the downwards movement closer to the spine and then move outwards once completed each parallel line (see image 64). Ensure the area is lubricated if you scrape directly on your skin.

ON YOUR ARMS

For puffy eyes, add the following:

5. Wide stroke down the Lung (LU) and up the Large intestine (LI) channels on your arm, especially on the muscle area before and after your elbow (see images 65-68). Repeat several times.

For crow's feet and puffy eyes, add the following:

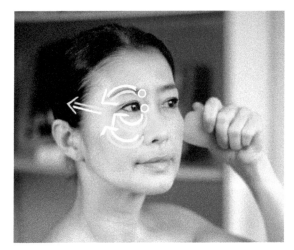

Image 63: Eye Step 1, 2 & 3

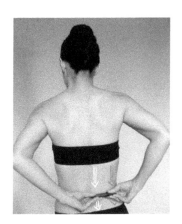
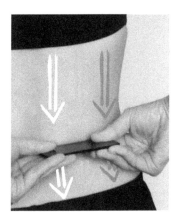

Image 64: Eye Step 4

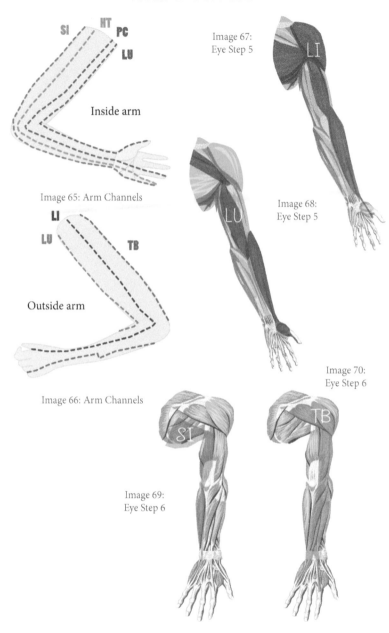

SI HT PC
LU

Inside arm

Image 65: Arm Channels

LI
LU   TB

Outside arm

Image 66: Arm Channels

Image 67:
Eye Step 5

LI

Image 68:
Eye Step 5

LU

Image 70:
Eye Step 6

Image 69:
Eye Step 6

SI   TB

6. Wide stroke up the muscles on the outside of your arm - the Small intestine (SI) and Triple burner (TB) channels (see images 65 and 66). On the upper arm, the triceps muscles at the back and on the lower arm the three main muscles which cover the watch side of your forearm (the extensor digiti minimi, extensor carpi ulnaris and flexor carpi ulnaris). Do not stroke on any bony areas or on the elbow itself (see images 69 and 70 for the muscle areas). Repeat several times.

ON YOUR LEGS

For dark rings under your eyes, follow 1, 2, 3, 4 and add:

7. Wide stroke up the Kidney (KD) and down the Bladder (BL) primary channels at the back of your legs (see image 71 and 72). It is often easier to follow the TM muscle groups as shown in images 73 and 74. Focus on the meaty upper muscles – the gastrocnemius/ soleus (calf muscles) and the biceps femoris/semitendinosus (thigh muscles). Ensure you have sufficient lubrication if scraping directly on your skin and repeat several times.

For puffy eyes, follow 1, 2, 3, 5, 6 and add:

8. Wide stroke up the Spleen (SP) and down the Stomach (ST) channels in your upper and lower leg (see images 71 and 72). As above, you do not need to narrowly follow the line of the primary channels, instead you should ensure that you cover the muscle groups that the channels pass through in that area. For the Stomach - the tibialis muscle on the outside of your lower leg and the big rectus femoris and vastus lateralis muscles on your thigh; for the Spleen, the flexor digitorum longus on the inside of your lower leg and the vastus medius and the sartorius on your inner thigh. This means that you are treating both the channels and the TM channels at the same time (see image 75 and 76). Ensure you have sufficient lubrication if scraping directly on your skin and repeat several times.

For crow's feet, follow 1, 2, 3, 6 and add:

9. Wide stroke down the Gall bladder (GB) and up the Liver (LV) channels in your upper and lower leg (see images 71 and 72). As above, make

Outside leg

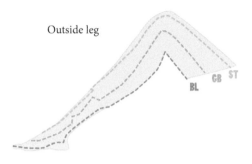

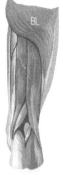

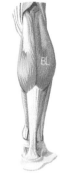

Image 71: Leg Channels

Image 73: Eye Step 7

Inside leg

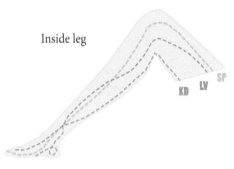

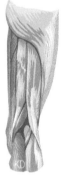

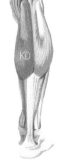

Image 72: Leg Channels

Image 74: Eye Step 7

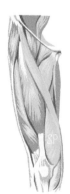

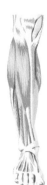

Image 75:
Eye Step 8

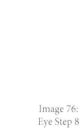

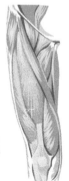

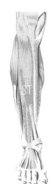

Image 76:
Eye Step 8

sure that you also cover the muscle groups as you go along the primary channels. For the Gall bladder – the peroneus tertius on the outside of the lower leg and the iliotibial tract and biceps femoris on the outside of your thigh; for the Liver – the extensor halluces longus in the front of your lower leg and the gracilis on the inside of your thigh (see images 77 and 78). Ensure you have sufficient lubrication if scraping directly on your skin and repeat several times.

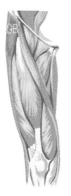
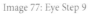
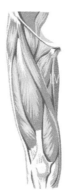

Image 77: Eye Step 9   Image 78: Eye Step 9

3. NOSE AREA

COMMON AGING FEATURES

Bunny lines

MUSCLES AND TISSUES

Ironically one of the side effects of chemical over treatment in removing wrinkles on your face is actually more pronounced transverse lines at the side of the nose. These are especially noticeable when you smile, causing the nasalis (G) and levator labii superioris alaeque nasi (H) muscles to contract (see image 79).

Scrunch your nose and notice the lines created at the side of the nose. Now relax your nose and see if those lines have disappeared. If they are still there, they are known as rhytids along the lateral nasal wall or simply as 'bunny lines'.

The levator labii alaeque superioris nasi muscle (H) dilates your nostrils and lifts your upper lip. Its origin is the upper part of your maxilla bone and its insertion is the side of your nostril and upper lip. The nasalis mainly works by opening your nostrils and is located closer to the actual side of your nose.

Apart from a side effect of too many Botox injections, repetitive movements of these muscles along with the lateral part of the orbicularis oculi muscle (C) are thought to be the cause.

CHANNELS AND POINTS

○ Like so many of the muscles in the face, the levator labii superioris alaeque nasi and the nasalis muscles are part of the Stomach TM channel. This means that distal treatment along the Stomach TM channel in the muscles of your legs will have an effect on the musculature this area.

○ While no primary channels pass directly through this area, both the Bladder and Large intestine primary channels connect to the ends of the muscles (see image 79).

○ The origin of both muscles lies close to Bl-1 (Bright eyes) which is just above the inside of your eye (see image 79). As its name suggests it is usually connected to treatment of your eyes and is featured in the previous section.

○ Bitong is an extra point, not connected to any channels, which lies mid-way along the levator labii superioris alaeque nasi muscle and affects your nose, nostrils and breathing.

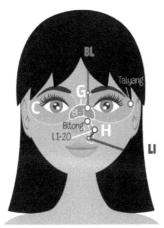

Image 79: Nose muscles, channels and points

You can find it where the flare of your nostrils ends on the nose (see image 79).

○ The insertion of these muscles is very close to Large Intestine 20 (Welcome fragrance) which is next to the midpoint of the flare of the nostrils. This point also influences your nose and breathing and is the last point on the Large intestine channel (LI) (see image 79).

NOSE SEQUENCE

ON YOUR FACE

1. Static circle for 5 seconds at LI-20 at the side of the flare of your nostrils and Bitong, slightly above and more towards your nose (see image 80).

2. Sweep up with the long side of your tool from LI-20. Go beside your nose and lift up to below your eye.

3. Gently static circle Bl-1 to the nose side of your eye socket for 5 seconds. Do not circle any soft tissue around your eye, only the bony area where your eye socket meets your nose.

4. Sweep across your eye socket to the temple area.

5. Static circle at Taiyang, an extra point at your temple, for 5 seconds.

6. Continue the sweeping movement above your ear and then down behind the ear to the neck.

Repeat the sequence three to five times.

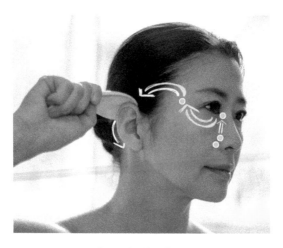

Image 80: Nose Steps 1-6

ON YOUR ARMS

7. Wide stroke up the Large intestine (LI) primary channel in your arm. Imagine that the elbow crease represents your eye level and that your wrist crease is your chin. You can then locate the approximate position of your nose along your arm (see image 81 and 82). Ensure you have sufficient lubrication if scraping directly on your skin and repeat several times.

ON YOUR LEGS

8. Wide stroke down the Stomach (ST) and Bladder (BL) primary channels in your lower leg (see image 83). Imagine that the knee crease represents your eye level and that your ankle bone is your chin. You can then locate the approximate position of your nose along the channel. See images 84 and 85 for details of muscles. Ensure you have sufficient lubrication if scraping directly on your skin and repeat several times.

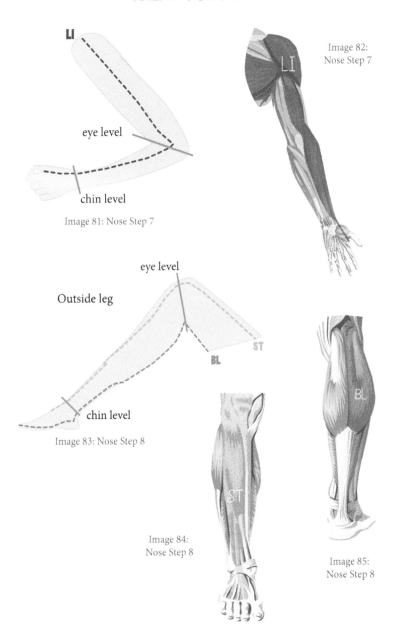

LI

eye level

chin level

Image 81: Nose Step 7

Image 82:
Nose Step 7

LI

eye level

Outside leg

ST

BL

chin level

Image 83: Nose Step 8

BL

ST

Image 84:
Nose Step 8

Image 85:
Nose Step 8

4. CHEEK AND MOUTH AREA

Your lips, mouth and surrounding soft-tissue are key in how we communicate non-verbally, at least in Western cultures. We smile, laugh, grin, grimace, sneer, bare our teeth, stick out our tongue and have all sorts of messages which are displayed from our mouth area. Having lived in Japan, I know that not all cultures share this toothy display of emotion (for Japan, it is the eyes) but our fixation with the mouth area and any visible signs of aging in this area can really affect how you see yourself and your self-confidence in interpersonal relationships.

COMMON AGING FEATURES

Loss of facial volume, nasolabial folds or smile lines, vertical lip lines

MUSCLES AND TISSUES

FACIAL VOLUME LOSS

Your cheek is actually made up of a fat pad which is held in place by a combination of taught zygomatic ligaments and a soft tissue support structure (the SMAS as described earlier in the book). Over time, both of these weaken and your cheeks start to

display a hollowed-out look and the fat that was held tight is allowed to descend to create saggy cheeks.

NASOLABIAL FOLDS

This can then lead on to the deepening of nasolabial folds or 'smile lines'. These are the lines which run from the side of your nose to the side of your mouth. As you age (from your third decade onwards) they can become more distinct because the collagen and elastin fibres in the connective tissue gradually break down and this reduces the skin's ability to spring back into shape.

This is especially so with these lines because they mark the dramatic boundary between two distinct areas of the face: the superficial tissues of the upper lip area which are firmly held in place by tightly connected muscle and skin, and the cheek fascia which is loose and spread over a wide area.

In general, if the upper part of the line is deeper, it suggests that emotions such as disgust or anger may be prominent in creating them. If however it is the lower part which is deeper, emotions connected to grief, sadness and

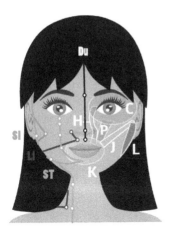

Image 86: Cheek Muscles & Channels

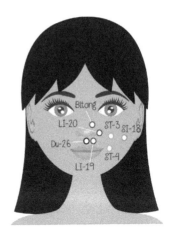

Image 87: Cheek Points

joy may be more involved. This is because of the repetitive nature of the muscle movement used when expressing these emotions.

There are two important muscles which affect nasolabial folds.

○ The levator labii superioris (P) lifts your upper lip (see image 86). It originates at your lower orbit and goes down to insert into the top of your lip. It is the movement of this muscle that affects the middle portion of the nasolabial fold.

○ The other important muscle is the levator labii superioris alaeque nasi (H) which splits into two as it descends from the maxilla bone, one part blends into your nose and the other merges into your upper lip with the levator labii superioris (see image 86). It acts by lifting your upper lip and flaring your nostrils to create a snarl. For this reason it is connected to the upper part of the fold.

VERTICAL LIP LINES

Vertical lines known as rhytids above your top lip have already been mentioned regarding smoking as they are classic skin feature of a long-term smoker. But you do not have to smoke in order to have them.

As you get older, the skin between your nose and top lip loses its elasticity and can become stretched and baggy. There is less subcutaneous tissue around your mouth with age and this combined with repetitive muscle actions which bunch the skin and soft-tissue together can cause visible lines.

The underlying muscle is the orbicularis oris (K) muscle, a circular muscle around your mouth which helps you to open and close it (see image 86).

These lines are less common in men due to the abundance of hair follicles and sweat glands in this area which give added structure to the tissue.

CHANNELS AND POINTS

FACIAL VOLUME LOSS

The two key primary channels which affect the cheek and mouth area are the Large intestine (LI) and the Stomach (ST) and this can clearly be seen from the trajectories of these channels (see image 86). The Small intestine channel (SI), however, also passes over your cheek and SI-18 (Cheek Bone Crevice) is below your cheek bone, level with the outside of your eye (see image 87). It is a point often used to affect the facial muscles in this area and lies between the masseter (L) and zygomaticus major (J) muscles which run across your cheek to your mouth.

NASOLABIAL FOLDS

The very last point on the Large intestine primary channel, LI-20 (Welcome Fragrance), is actually at the start of the nasolabial fold at the flare of the nostrils (see image 87). It is also the meeting point with the Stomach channel and just below Bitong, an extra point next to your nose and which lies within the levator labii superioris alaeque nasi muscle (H).

ST-4 (Earth Granary) is located at the other end of the nasolabial fold at the side of your mouth. It is located actually in the nasolabial groove (see image 87) and is mainly used to treat disorders of your facial muscles. Below ST-4 in the body of the depressor anguli oris muscle is the motor nerve insertion. ST-3 (Great Crevice) is also located at the origin of the levator labii superioris muscle (P) at the zygomatic bone.

VERTICAL LIP LINES

The Large intestine primary channel passes through the area between your upper lip and nose. LI-19 (Mouth Grain Crevice) is below your nostril, directly over the insertion of the motor nerve in the muscle belly of the orbicularis oris, a muscle which is actually part of the long Stomach TM channel (see image 87).

The Du channel ends at Du-26 (Water Trough) on the midline of the philtrum between your mouth and nose. It is an important point for treatment because it is the meeting point of the Large intestine and Stomach channels (see image 87).

MOUTH/CHEEK AREA SEQUENCE

ON YOUR FACE

The following sequences will benefit both loss of facial volume and nasolabial folds.

1. Static circle at Bitong at the side of your nose for five seconds. Then sweep across your face below your cheek bone up to your temple area. The sweep is one movement gently pulling at the muscle fibres below (see image 88).

2. Static circle at LI-20 for five seconds. Then sweep across the middle of your cheek (over ST-3, the origin of the levator labii superioris alaeque nasi muscle) and then up to the temple area (see image 88).

3. Static circle at ST-4 at the side of your mouth for five seconds. Then sweep across the lower part of your cheek and then up to the temple area (see image 88).

4. Put the (longer) side of the tool at a 45 degree angle along the nasolabial fold. Slide it up the side of your nose to just below your eye. Then sweep across following under your cheek bone (not your eye socket) to the front of your ear. Continue the movement over the ear and then down the side of your neck. The whole thing is one smooth movement. Repeat three to five times (see image 89).

5. Corner circle at Du-26 below the centre of your nose and then sweep across the area above your lip to ST-4 at side of your mouth. After you reach ST-4, sweep up below your cheek bone to your temple (see image 90).

6. Repeat this below your mouth. Static circle at Ren-24 and sweep across below your lip to ST-4. Then sweep up to your temple (see image 90).

81

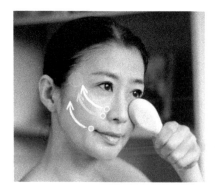

Image 88: Cheek Steps 1-3

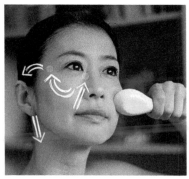

Image 89: Cheek Step 4

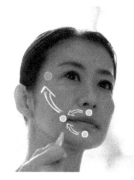

Image 90: Cheek Steps 5-6

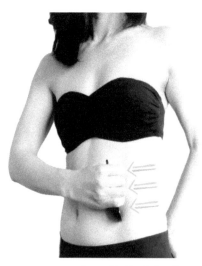

Image 91: Cheek Step 7

Inside leg

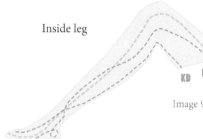

Image 93: Cheek Step 9

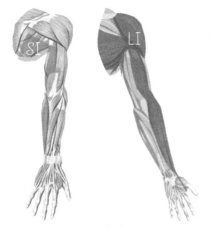

Image 92: Cheek Step 8

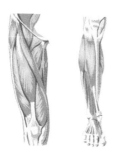

Image 94: Cheek Step 9

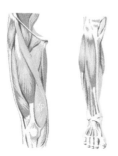

Image 95: Cheek Step 9

ON YOUR BODY

7. Sweep across your abdomen both above and below your belly button. The strokes should be gentle with the idea of both crossing the Stomach, Spleen and Kidney primary channels and also to firm the muscles in this area (see image 91). This technique is ideal if you have more fatty tissue in this area than you would like! Repeat several times and ensure the skin is sufficiently lubricated.

ON YOUR ARMS

8. Wide stroke up the muscles of the Large intestine (LI) and Small intestine (SI) TM channels on the lower and upper arm, especially the area below and above your elbow (see image 92). Repeat several times.

ON YOUR LEGS

9. Wide stroke up the Spleen (SP) and Liver (LV) primary/ TM channels on the inside of your lower and upper leg. The Liver channel will affect the Large intestine and Small intestine channels and the Spleen channel affects the Stomach and Small intestine channels (see image 93, 94, 95). Repeat several times.

5. LOWER FACE AND NECK AREA

COMMON AGING FEATURES

Double chin, marionette lines, jowls, platysmal banding

MUSCLES AND TISSUES

As you age, your lower face and neck area is affected by changes in fat deposits and sagging jowls, vertical lines on the neck known as platysmal banding and the reabsorption of part of the jaw bone and chin. These changes often mean the loss of contour of your jawline and less of a demarcation between where your face ends and neck begins.

LOWER FACE FOLDS

These are short vertical lines that descend from the corners of your mouth known as marionette lines and commissural lines. They often accompany deep nasolabial folds as featured in the previous section. They appear very much like many of the other facial features of aging due to muscle hyperactivity and loss of elasticity. The key muscles being the depressor anguli oris (I) and platysma muscles (Q) which pull your mouth downwards (see image 96).

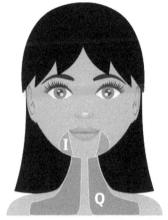

Image 96: Face and neck muscles

JOWLS

With the loss of muscular tension, there develops an accumulation of fat in your lower cheek which overlaps your mandible (lower jaw bone). This fat has been shifted downwards due to tissue volume loss, gravity and physical changes in the mandible bone.

SAGGING CHIN

As muscles begin to loosen and your skin loses its tone and elasticity, the chances of developing a sagging or double chin increases. This is partly because your maxilla (upper jaw bone) and mandible (lower jawbone) lose their bone density and your face can appear slightly shorter and wider as you get older.

Also under the midline of your chin there is usually an accumulation of subcutaneous fat and it is these fat deposits which become more pronounced through weight gain and aging.

PLATYSMAL BANDS

Below this fat layer in your neck is the platysma muscle (Q), a thin sheet of muscle originating from fascia and skin over the pectoral (chest) and deltoid (shoulder) muscles. There is a platysma muscle on each side of your neck and when it passes over your jawbone it changes into collagen fibres and connective tissue and blends into the skin on your face. It pulls your lower lip and the corner of your mouth to the side and downwards, opening your mouth, often to express surprise or fright.

As we get older, this muscle starts to lose its tone and becomes stretched. This causes the muscle fibres to bind together and become visible as 'bands' either side of your neck.

CHANNELS AND POINTS

LOWER FACE FOLDS

The Stomach primary channel and the Bladder and Large intestine TM channels pass through the lower face and neck and have a strong influence over the tissue and muscles of this area. The two key muscles in lower face folds are part of different channels: the depressor anguli oris is part of the Large intestine TM channel and the platysma muscles are part of the Bladder TM channel. The Stomach primary channel slices horizontally through both (see image 97).

There are also two points below your mouth which are usually stimulated to affect the Kidney and lower back problems. Shui Tong (Water Through) is below the corner of your mouth and Shui Jin (Water Metal) is to the side of the midline below your mouth. This area can sometimes be slightly darker than the skin around it and have spider veins if there is lower back pain (see image 97).

JOWLS

As the presence of jowls usually means the loosening and descending of tissue from above, much of what was mentioned in facial volume loss in the previous section applies here. The Stomach primary channel runs from your chin along your mandible bone to the angle of your jaw and then makes a 90 degree turn upwards through your temple to the corner of your head. This part of the channel includes ST-5 (Great Welcome) in front of the masseter muscle, ST-6 (Jaw bone) at the angle of the jaw in the head of the masseter muscle and ST-7 (Below the joint) in line with the middle of your ear and a meeting point of the Stomach and Gall Bladder channels (see image 97). All of these points have traditionally been associated with local treatment of the mouth, jaw, teeth and cheek.

SAGGING CHIN

The two primary channels which pass through the area of a double chin are Stomach (ST) and Ren. The Stomach channel descends down the side of the laryngeal prominence (Adam's apple) towards your clavicle bone and the Ren channel is heading in the opposite direction upwards on the centreline and finishes at Ren-24 (Container of Fluids), in the midline gap between the orbicularis oris and the two mentalis muscles below your bottom lip.

The development of a double chin is traditionally connected with the function of your kidneys in Oriental Medicine but what the ancient Chinese were referring to is not actually your kidneys but your adrenal glands which sit on top of your kidneys. The hormonal imbalance that can be created when these glands under

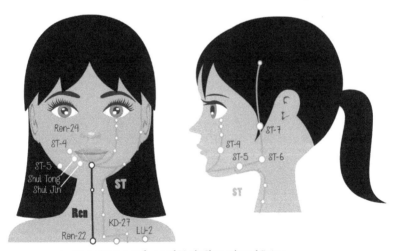

Image 97: Lower face and Neck Channels and Points

or over-perform can lead to an accumulation of subcutaneous fat under your chin.

PLATYSMAL BANDS

The platysma muscles are part of the Bladder TM channel which mostly covers the back of your body apart from your neck and face. The sternocleidomastoid and trapezius muscles which cover the sides and back of your neck make up the rest of the Bladder TM channel of the neck so treatment on these will have a knock on effect to the platysma muscles.

The origin of the platysma muscle also covers the beginning of the Lung primary channel at LU-2 and the end of the Kidney primary channel at KD-27. In order to affect changes to the origin of the muscle, both the Kidney and Lung channels are obvious candidates both locally and distally.

LOWER FACE/NECK AREA SEQUENCE

The following sequences will benefit your lower face and neck:

ON YOUR FACE

1. Static circle at Ren-24 for five seconds and sweep across below your lip to ST-4. Then sweep up to your temple. Do this three times and then repeat this on the other side of your face (see image 98).

2. Sweep horizontally across from Ren-24 just above your mandible bone. Static circle at ST-5 for five seconds, at the edge of the masseter muscle, and then continue to sweep until ST-6 at the angle of the jaw. Static circle here for five seconds and then switch the tool to its widest side and

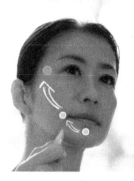

Image 98: Lower face Step 1

sweep up your cheek following the Stomach primary channel to your temple area (see image 99).

3. Use the concave part in tool if there is one and place the tool under the centre of the chin. Press for a few seconds and

87

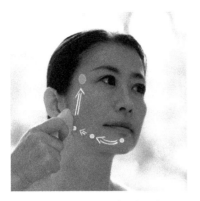

Image 99: Lower face Step 2

then slide along the edge of the mandible bone. If there is no concave part to your tool, use the flatter side. As you reach the end of the mandible, bring the side of the tool flat on to the skin and slide it under your ear and then down the side of your neck. Repeat this three to five times (see image 100).

ON YOUR NECK

4. Tilt your head backwards and sweep downwards under your chin and neck. Cover the whole chin/jaw/neck area but be careful not to stroke onto the laryngeal prominence (Adam's apple) and be aware of the presence of lymph nodes and the carotid arteries between the sternocleido-mastoid muscle and trachea (windpipe). Repeat this three to five times. If having Gua sha petechiae marks on your neck is acceptable, you can use a wide stroke technique, especially if you your neck is prone to stiffness as this should make it feel less stiff (see image 101). Repeat several times.

5. Scrape down the muscles of the back of your neck. Start at your occiput and wide stroke downwards following vertical lines across your neck. Be careful of your vertebrae at the centreline. You can scrape down on the bone if there is sufficient soft tissue to act as a cushion but be cautious especially if you have any structural neck issues (see image 102). Repeat several times.

ON YOUR SHOULDER

6. Wide stroke over your trapezius shoulder muscle down towards your arm. The trapezius is part of the Bladder TM channel (see image 103). Repeat several times.

7. Wide stroke over the deltoid muscle on the side of your shoulder/top of your arm. This is a part of the Large intestine TM channel. Avoid scraping over the acromion

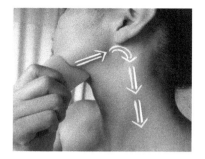

Image 100: Neck Step 3

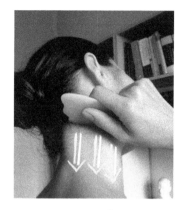

Image 101: Neck Step 4

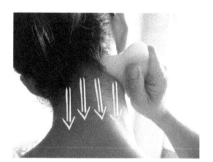

Image 102: Neck Step 5

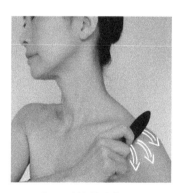

Image 104: Neck Step 7

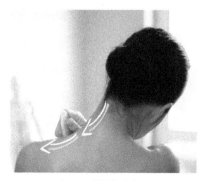

Image 103: Neck Step 6

bone (see image 104). Repeat several times.

ON YOUR CHEST

8. Narrow stroke from the midline outwards in the tissue above your clavicle bone (not on the bone). Then repeat below the bone (see image 105). This technique can produce petechiae marks on your skin.

9. Narrow stroke across the top area of your chest. Start at your sternum and stroke across following the curved gaps in your rib cage. Avoid stroking directly on your ribs or on breast tissue (see image 105). Repeat several times.

ON YOUR ARMS

10. Wide stroke down the Lung (LU) primary/TM channel in your lower and upper arm (see images 106 and 107). Repeat several times.

ON YOUR LEGS

11. Wide stoke down the Stomach primary/TM channel in your lower and upper leg (see images 108 and 109). Repeat several times.

12. Wide stoke up the Kidney primary/TM channel in your lower and upper leg (see image 110 and 111). Repeat several times.

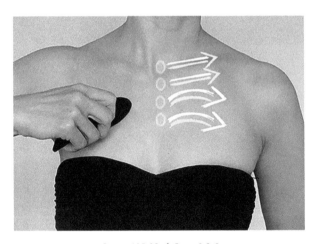

Image 105: Neck Steps 8 & 9

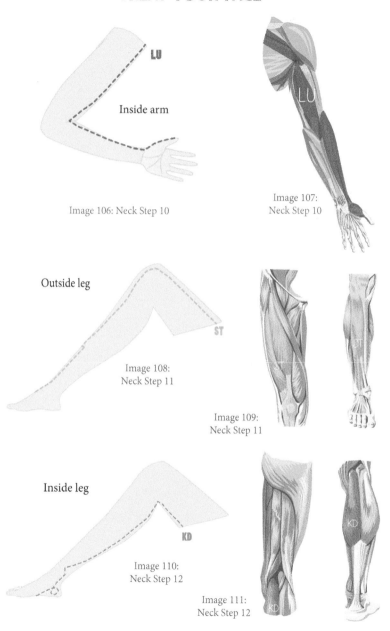

LU

Inside arm

LU

Image 106: Neck Step 10

Image 107:
Neck Step 10

Outside leg

ST

Image 108:
Neck Step 11

Image 109:
Neck Step 11

Inside leg

KD

Image 110:
Neck Step 12

Image 111:
Neck Step 12

PUTTING IT ALL TOGETHER

COMBINE THE SEQUENCES

The key to effective treatment is to combine the Gua sha sequences so that they address what matters to you. If you wish to treat your whole face, you can put the individual sequences into one long sequence. If you wish to target certain areas, well, hopefully you now have the knowledge and tools to do this and to create your own sequence.

Here is an example sequence which uses your whole body to treat your face both locally and distally:

A. LOOSEN

1. Loosen your head
Follow the instructions as detailed on p.47-9 for relaxing the head area.

2. Loosen your face
Follow the instructions as detailed on p.49-51 for relaxing the face area.

○ HEAD

3. Forehead Step 5 (see image 112-3) Instructions on p.57

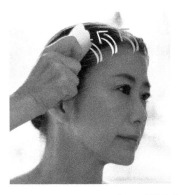 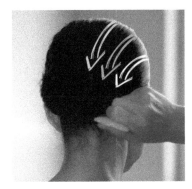

Image 112-3: Forehead Step 5

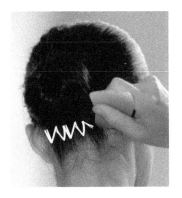

4. Forehead Step 6 (see image 114) Instructions on p.57-8

Image 114: Forehead Step 6

○ FACE

5. Forehead Steps 1-3 (see image 115). Instructions on p.56-7

Image 115: Forehead Steps 1-3

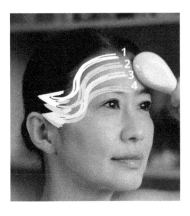

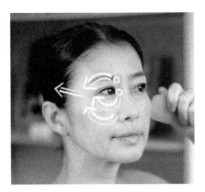

Image 116: Eye Steps 1-3

6. Eye steps 1-3 (see image 116) Instructions on p.68

7. Nose steps 1-5 (see image 117) Instructions on p.75

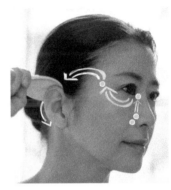

Image 117: Nose Steps 1-5

8. Cheek Steps 1-3 (see image 118) Instructions on p.81

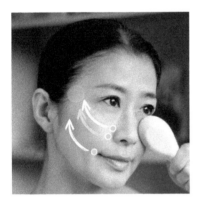

Image 118: Cheek Steps 1-3

9. Cheek Step 4 (see image 119) Instructions on p.81

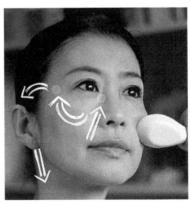

Image 119: Cheek Step 4

10. Cheek Step 5-6 (see image 120)
Instructions on p.81

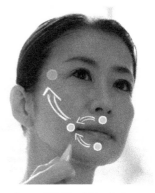

Image 120: Cheek Step 5-6

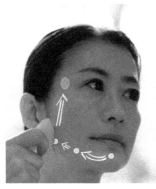

Image 121: Lower face Step 2

11. Lower face Step 2 (see image 121) Instructions on p.87

12. Neck Step 3 (see image 122) Instructions on p.87

○ NECK

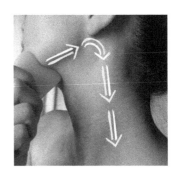

Image 122: Neck Step 3

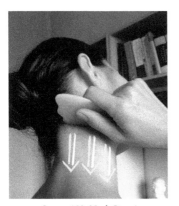

Image 123: Neck Step 4

13. Neck Step 4 (see image 123) Instructions on p.88

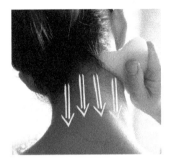

Image 124: Neck Step 5

14. Neck Step 5 (see image 124)
Instructions on p.88

o SHOULDERS

15. Neck Step 6 (see image 125)
Instructions on p.88

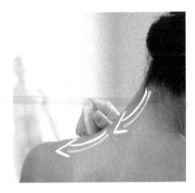

Image 125: Neck Step 6

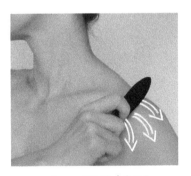

Image 126: Neck Step 7

16. Neck Step 7 (see image 126)
Instructions on p.88-90

o CHEST

17. Neck Step 8-9 (see image 127)
Instructions on p.90

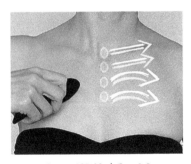

Image 127: Neck Step 8-9

PUTTING IT ALL TOGETHER

○ LOWER BACK

18. Eye Step 4 (see image 128)
Instructions on p.68

○ WAIST

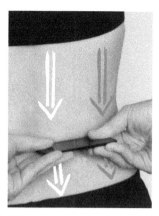

Image 128: Eye Step 4

19. Forehead Step 7 (see image
129) Instructions on p.58

○ ABDOMEN

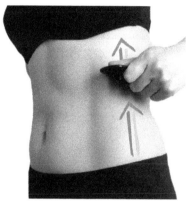

Image 129: Forehead Step 7

20. Cheek Step 7 (see image 130)
Instructions on p.83

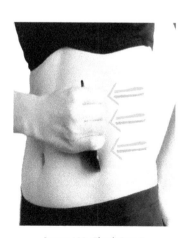

Image 130: Cheek Step 7

○ ARMS   Image 131: Forehead Steps 8-9 & Eye step 5

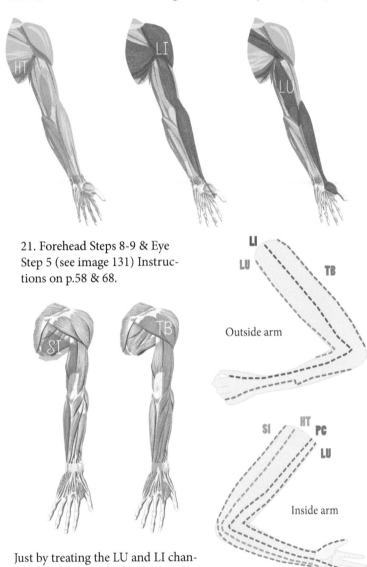

21. Forehead Steps 8-9 & Eye
Step 5 (see image 131) Instructions on p.58 & 68.

Just by treating the LU and LI channels you can cover all the areas of
your face.

98

O LEGS   22. Eye Steps 7-9 (see image 132) Instructions on p.71-3.

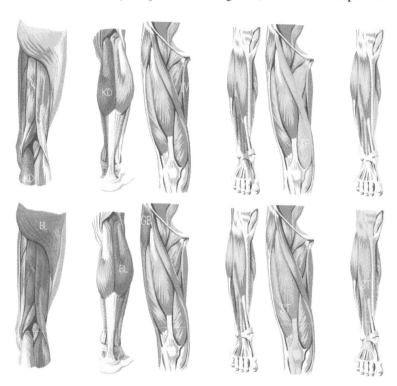

Image 132: Eye Steps 7-9

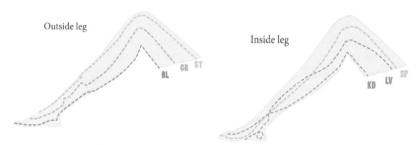

Outside leg

Inside leg

Just by treating the ST and LV channels you can cover all the areas of your face.

EXPECTATIONS

In our world of instant grati-
fication, impatience is very much
endemic. We want our issues
dealt with now. I send a message
across the planet and get a reply
before I have even taken a sip of
my coffee. I browse online in the
early hours of the morning and
buy my weekly shopping with a
click. I can see what my friends
get up to in real time on social
networks. Our expectations are
instant because technology has
created the possibility. The problem is that this spills over to other
areas of life where such expectations are more unreasonable.

I run an acupuncture clinic
in a Spanish enclave in North
Africa (yep, it is a long story),
and patients often come in with
these expectations. If you have
had a chronic health issue for
20 years, it will not normally get
better after one treatment, or
two or three or ten. In fact, the
standard rule of thumb for this
type of acupuncture treatment is
that for every year you have had
the problem, it will take a month
of treatment to resolve it. As you
might guess, this is not what most
people want to hear. They want
a quick fix for something that
took a lifetime to create. This is
of course the draw of plastic surgery. The nip and tuck culture of
cosmetic 'procedures' fits the bill
perfectly. Why let nature take its
course when you can nip nature
in the bud and slice, stretch, pull,
suck and freeze your way to a new
face. In fact why wait. You can
even have it done in your lunch
hour.

SEQUENCE FREQUENCY

I hope that this book has
gone some way in explaining why
this short-term fix may not last
long. Your face has its own ideas
about how it should look based
on your lifestyle, diet, emotional
stress etc. and it will return to
that state as long as you neglect
to see the whole picture of how
it is connected to the health of
your body. If you are focused on
making changes on this connective basis, do not expect an
overnight miracle with one or two
sequence repetitions. Of course,
you should see subtle changes
right away as the increased blood
circulation passes through tissue
and muscle and for some this may
appear much more dramatic but
for sustained, real changes you
have to repeat the sequences on a
regular basis. Three times a week
is a good start. Any less than this
and you will not see the consistent results. And dare I say it. You
need a little patience. Think in

terms of weeks and months. You have to remember that the aim is for changes in the face through your body as well as your face so you need to give it a chance to work.

ENJOY THE SEQUENCES

Do not get too hung up on the channels, points and muscles. They have been included here to give you the full background so that you can understand that when I suggest scraping in a particular area, I am not pulling the ideas out of thin air but basing them on solid theories in Oriental medicine and established anatomical locations. How much you want to go into this is your choice, you can just skip it if you prefer and go straight into the sequences. Changes in your face are not dependent on you understanding what is happening. Those changes will happen anyway. You just need to follow the sequences. So relax. Enjoy. And get stroking.

MORE INFORMATION

For more information and videos on Gua sha, please visit www.clivewitham.com. You can also find information on Facebook at https://www.facebook.com/WorldofOM/ or contact me directly at clive@medicinaoriental.org if you have any queries and I will do my best to answer them.

ENDNOTES

1. ISAPS, 2015. International Survey on Aesthetic/Cosmetic Procedures Performed in 2014. International Society of Aesthetic Plastic Surgery.

2. VAN ARSDALL, A. 2016. Herbs and Healers from the Ancient Mediterranean. Through the Medieval West: Essays in Honor of John M.Riddle. Routledge.

3. MIN LING. 2012. Research on Cosmetology of Traditional Chinese Medicine. Chapter 56 Informatics and Management Science IV Volume 207 of the series Lecture Notes in Electrical Engineering pp 457-462

4. ZHANG, D and YONG XU, F. 2016. Computer Models for Facial Beauty Analysis. Springer.

5. PERON, A et al. 2012. Photometric study of divine proportion and its correlation with facial attractiveness. Dental Press J Orthod. Mar-Apr;17 (2):124-31.

6. North American Caucasians: Revision of Neoclassical Canons. Plastic & Reconstructive Surgery: March, Volume 75,Issue 3, ppg 328-337.

7. LI ZHIXIN. 2011. Fight aging, blemishes with guasha facial. Beijing Today, May 27.

8. NIELSEN,A. Gua Sha: A Traditional Technique for Modern Practice. New York: Churchill Livingstone, 2013.

9. QIN-YAN XU et al. 2012. "The Effects of Scraping Therapy on Local Temperature and Blood Perfusion Volume in Healthy Subjects," Evidence-Based Complementary and Alternative Medicine.

10. Y. Y. WANG, W. J. YI, AND W. L. LIU. 2009. "Brief introduction to the functions of points in scraping therapy. Report at 2009 Annual Conference sponsored by China Association of Acupuncture and Moxibustion," Bian stone Forum, pp. 138–139.

11. MIN LING. Chapter 56 Research on Cosmetology of Traditional Chinese Medicine in W. DU (ed.). 2013. Informatics and Management Science IV, Lecture Notes in Electrical Engineering 207

12. BRIDGES, L. 2004. Face Reading in Chinese Medicine. St. Louis: Churchill Livingstone.

13. DOSHI DN, HANNEMAN KK, COOPER KD. 2007. Smoking and skin aging in identical twins. Arch Dermatol; 143: 1543–1546.

14. MODEL D. 1985. Smoker's face: an underrated clinical sign? Br Med J (Clin Res Ed); 291: 1760–1762.

15. DANBY FW. 2011. Acne: Diet and acnegenesis. Indian Dermatology Online Journal; 2(1):2-5. doi:10.4103/2229-5178.79851.

16. CRANE JD et al. 2015. Exercise-stimulated interleukin-15 is controlled by AMPK and regulates skin metabolism and aging. Aging Cell, 14: 625–634. doi:10.1111/acel.1234.

17. UNIVERSITY OF ST ANDREWS. 2010. Growing old gracefully.14 September. Available at https://www.st-andrews.ac.uk/news/archive/2010/title,55666,en.php.

18. MEADOWS, G. 2015. Jodie Kidd reveals the shocking impact sleep deprivation can have on our skin. May 18. Available at http://www.bensonsforbeds.co.uk/sleep-school/does-sleep-deprivation-effect-our-appearance/#_ftnref1

19. BURGESS JA et al. 2009. Does eczema lead to asthma? J Asthma. Jun;46(5):429-36. doi: 10.1080/02770900902846356.

20. LI X, KONG L, LI F, CHEN C, XU R, et al. 2015. Association between Psoriasis and Chronic Obstructive Pulmonary Disease: A Systematic Review and Meta-analysis. PLOS ONE 10(12): e0145221. https://doi.org/10.1371/journal.pone.0145221

21. LEWIS MB, BOWLER PJ. 2009. Botulinum toxin cosmetic therapy correlates with a more positive mood. J Cosmet Dermatol., 8, 24-6.

22. J. S. XU, et al. 2010. "Effects of electroacupuncture on microcirculation perfusion and infrared radiation track of the body surface," Fujian TCM College, vol. 20, no. 1, pp. 13–15.

23. NGUYEN HT, ISAACOWITZ, DM, RUBIN, PA. 2009. Age- and fatigue-related markers of human faces: an eye-tracking study. Ophthalmology.116 (2):355–60.

INDEX